Ethics in Nursing
The Caring Relationship

Verena Tschudin RGN RM DipCouns BSc(Hons) MA PhD
University of Surrey, UK

THIRD EDITION

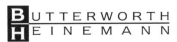

BUTTERWORTH
HEINEMANN
An Imprint of Elsevier Science

EDINBURGH LONDON NEW YORK OXFORD PHILADELPHIA
ST LOUIS SYDNEY TORONTO 2002

BUTTERWORTH-HEINEMANN
An imprint of Elsevier Science Limited

First edition 1986
Second edition 1992
Revised reprint 1993
Third edition 2003

ISBN 0 7506 5265 9

British Library Cataloguing in Publication Data
A catalogue record for this book is available from the British Library

Library of Congress Cataloging in Publication Data
A catalog record for this book is available from the Library of Congress

Note
Medical knowledge is constantly changing. As new information
becomes available, changes in treatment, procedures, equipment and
the use of drugs become necessary. The author and the publishers have
taken care to ensure that the information given in this text is accurate
and up to date. However, readers are strongly advised to confirm that
the information, especially with regard to drug usage, complies with
the latest legislation and standards of practice.

 ELSEVIER SCIENCE

your source for books,
journals and multimedia
in the health sciences

www.elsevierhealth.com

The
publisher's
policy is to use
**paper manufactured
from sustainable forests**

Printed in China by RDC Group Limited

Ethics in Nursing

This book is due for return on or before the last date shown

14 JUN 2003

I1

For Butterworth-Heinemann:

Commissioning Editor: Mary Seager
Development Editor: Catherine Jackson
Project Manager: Morven Dean
Design: George Ajayi

Contents

Preface to the third edition

Ethics will always produce more questions than satisfactory answers. Despite the tomes that have been written about it — this one included — there is never one answer, theory, principle or rule that can be applied directly to any situation. Perhaps this is just as well, as it highlights the wonderful diversity of human living and acting. Ethics is therefore above all a venture in how to be human.

Writing a book reveals much about an author. A new edition of a book may also reveal to the world how the author has changed in the time between the last edition and the present one, and this is certainly the case here. Indeed, the subject of ethics has changed a great deal, and so have I. In earlier editions I stressed the need to listen to and hear each other, and this has become of increasing concern to me. This stems from personal experience of not being heard, especially as a patient, and the realisation of the damage that this can cause. It stems also from considerable teaching experience, where listening to students and hearing their stories and concerns has resulted in some of the most significant learning for me. Much of the time, our students teach us more than we may be able to acknowledge or believe. Perhaps how we teach them may be as important as what we teach them. Certainly, how we are with patients is as important as what we do with or to them. At the interface lies our ethical being and thinking.

In the 1970s I trained as a counsellor and it was this that led me into ethics. It was counselling that made me acutely aware of the supremacy of the helping relationship. It is therefore as a counsellor that I work on ethics, and as a teacher and writer of ethics that I do my counselling. The two disciplines complement each other, which is clearly visible in this book. I am, however, not advocating that they are necessary to practise nursing generally.

This is a basic text about ethics, and one among many others.

My hope is that it will contribute to the general knowledge of this field. The companion volume, *Approaches to Ethics: Nursing Beyond Boundaries* should ideally be read alongside, as it gives an insight into how ethics can be broadened and applied in different ways, thus providing a wider perspective of its study and practice. Perhaps this is the most obvious way in which I have changed since writing the previous edition: I have gained an international perspective, and also learned about and worked with new and different approaches. My wish is that readers of both volumes will gain some nuggets of information from either or both volumes that may make their practice more ethical and therefore more satisfactory.

Verena Tschudin   London 2003

Acknowledgements

It is never possible to thank everyone who has contributed to a book. The printed text is only an end-product of much learning, reading, discussing and experiencing. Colleagues and students at the University of Surrey have contributed without being aware of it. Friends, and colleagues working with me on the journal *Nursing Ethics*, have certainly contributed in countless ways that enabled me to learn from them. I would like to thank them all. A special thank-you goes to Mary Seager at Elsevier, for persuading me to write this new edition, not taking no for an answer, and for being available at crucial moments. I am grateful to all members of the production team at Elsevier. Particular thanks go to Margaret Carver, a copy-editor colleague of many years, who took on this book. The people behind the scenes in publishing are the ones that make a book possible and it is they who deserve the bouquets.

1

Caring: a basis for ethics

THE UNIQUENESS OF CARING

Caring is not unique to nursing, but it is unique in nursing. Nursing is a practical hands-on job, where experience, emotion, affection and relationships make up the bulk of everyday work. Caring is about people. It is done with people, for people, to people and as people. It is this last aspect that makes caring unique: people relate to people; one person relates to another person.

AN ETHIC OF CARE

The first person to have used the expression 'ethic of care' is said to be Carol Gilligan (1982) in her well-known text *In a Different Voice*. She was quickly followed by many others, especially women and feminists, who realised that she was indeed saying something to which they could relate. Nursing, too, saw in an ethic of care a legitimate model to use. Sara Fry (1989) was an early protagonist, making a strong argument for a nursing ethic to be a feminine ethic, not bounded by the traditional 'masculine' principles. Patricia Benner and Judith Wrubel's book, *The Primacy of Caring*, was published in 1989, and Jean Watson and Marilyn Ray edited *The Ethics of Care and the Ethics of Cure* in 1990. Megan-Jane Johnstone (1994), too, was very clear that a nursing ethic is an ethic based on care and on feminine principles.

According to Nel Noddings (1984), an approach to ethics from caring is 'rooted in receptivity, relatedness, and responsiveness' (p. 2). Thus it is clear that the relationship between people, especially between nurses and patients, is so significant that a whole approach to ethical reasoning can be based on it.

Medical ethics had become established in the 1970s, mainly through the publication of *Principles of Biomedical Ethics* by Tom Beauchamp and James Childress, which is now it its fifth edition

(2001). This text was argued from principles first established by Hippocrates, in particular beneficence (doing good), non-maleficence (doing no harm), and justice. To these, Beauchamp and Childress added respect for autonomy. They were writing in an American context, where autonomy and individualism is very highly valued. These four basic principles came to be regarded as *the* principles for medicine and health care, and the term 'bioethics' came to be associated with them. Many nurses, in both the UK and the USA, used them without question, because nothing else was quite so authoritative or available. When feminist writers began to challenge these standard principles, labelling them as masculine, other approaches to health care ethics gradually emerged, and, today, 'principlism', as it has become known, is seriously challenged (DuBose et al 1994) as the only way to consider ethics within health care.

The principles of medical ethics do not necessarily fit nursing well, because the relationships between nurses and patients, and between doctors and patients, rest on different bases. Many practical and historical reasons account for this. The nurse–patient relationship remains one of more intimate and more long-term care. The relationship between doctor and patient is often characterised by an intermediary instrument: a stethoscope, a scalpel, or test results. These are usually the means for explanation or information and then the person withdraws. It is the nurses who are present when pain is experienced and expressed, when vulnerability is exposed, or when death approaches. These elements frequently demand a response rather than a technical or scientific response. They are thus the basis for an ethical approach to care, starting with receptivity, relatedness and responsiveness.

Any system of ethics demands critical reflection on the moral life. Johnstone (1994) wrote that 'ethical inquiry concerns itself not so much with how the world is, but rather with how it *ought* to be' (p. 39). Ethics asks and tries to identify what is good and right, bad and wrong. If one can take a principle, such as beneficence, and argue that 'doing good' in a situation means this or that, then everyone is happy. However, this is rarely the case, because what suits one person does not suit another. For one person, having an abortion is doing the right thing in a difficult situation, and for another person not having an abortion is the right thing to do. An ethic of care does not consider the principle in the first instance (i.e. doing right, or doing the right thing); it considers first the need of the person to be heard, accepted and responded to. The narrative the person presents is the basis for ethical decisions and actions.

In any situation of need or urgency, a person's value system, emotional needs, memories and 'gut feelings' play a large part. Many ethics systems rule out feelings and needs as unreliable, and want to make decisions entirely based on reason and rationality. No wonder that many people find it difficult to relate to them. For many, the heart rules the head, and this is the preferred way of making ethical decisions. An ethic of care takes this seriously and responds in ways that are adequate to the perceived needs. The need to 'care' is paramount. In this it is not just the 'cared-for' who benefits, but crucially also the 'one-caring' (Noddings 1984) in that the 'one-caring' is also receiving. In this way both parties are fulfilled and 'humanized'. This leads to that almost indefinable something that nurses know so well—and frequently describe as 'job satisfaction'—which is received when real caring happens.

Rita Manning (1998) describes five elements that constitute a care ethic: moral attention, sympathetic understanding, relationship awareness, accommodation and response. Such an ethic 'provides guidance about how to live our lives' (p. 105).

Moral attention to all the details of a situation is a basic need. This demands that care-givers have time and are able and willing to care in a holistic way.

Sympathetic understanding is close to what Carl Rogers (1961) calls 'unconditional positive regard' (p. 38), or the ability to see other persons and their world and being as this person sees them.

Relationship awareness is described in terms of three levels: the relationship we have as fellow creatures, the relationship of need and ability, and the relationship of professional and client or patient. All three are possible at any stage and all need to be taken into consideration.

Accommodation refers to considering everyone concerned. Every relationship involves other relationships. Here it means listening to all the people involved.

Response is the logical outcome of attention, understanding and the relationship. We become empowered to act according to what the person is, says, conveys, needs and possibly desires. The person has been heard.

Manning is clear that this approach to ethics is time consuming, and, in an increasingly specialised health care system, time is at a premium. In a setting where no-one has time, this in itself causes further ethical problems.

For these and other historical reasons, the ethic of care has not been accepted uncritically. Suzanne Gordon (1996) is very adamant that 'a significant group of feminists view the field of caring with deep suspicion' (p. 256). She argues that '[p]atriarchal societies have not truly valued caregiving, but have instead sentimentalized and romanticized what they insist are women's "superior moral virtues" and "natural" inclination to care for the dependent' (p. 257).

Helga Kuhse (1997), too, makes a strong point that an ethic of care is inadequate. The headings in her book give an indication of her position: 'Not all caring is good' (p. 153); 'Caring is arbitrary' (p. 154); 'Care knows no limits, no fairness and equality' (p. 159); and 'Silenced by care' (p. 161).

Joan Tronto (1993) argues that caring has always been done by less powerful people in society. She says that 'we come [close] to the reality when we say: caring about, and taking care of, are the duties of the powerful. Care-giving and care-receiving are left to the less powerful' (p. 114).

The terms 'caring', 'caring about' and 'taking care of' have come to be used as the criteria over which the pros and cons of an ethic of care are argued.

Tronto devotes large parts of her book to arguing that an ethic of care has its place, and indeed a legitimate place. Her book is subtitled 'A political argument for an ethic of care'. She sees the struggle as an ethic of care being both based in politics and needing a political defence. This accords well with Geoffrey Hunt's (1991) argument that 'there is a need for a shift in our conception of health care, and this entails a recognition not only of the wider social and economic construction of illness and health care but, from the moral point of view, a recognition of what is ineradicable and unchangeable in the human condition' (p. 18).

Hunt goes on to state that it may now be the turn of the nursing profession 'to lead health care out of the blind alley in which it has become trapped. This means turning health care the right way up – making treatment and cure subordinate to care' (p. 18).

Despite its shortcomings and the attacks made on it, an ethic of care within nursing is a useful and powerful way for considering ethics. No system is completely adequate or appropriate; an ethic of care within nursing is at least as, and in Hunt's argument perhaps more than, adequate than many others.

An ethic of care is firmly based on the relationship between the person caring and the person receiving care. Throughout this book, the caring relationship is the concern. It is not possible to say that an ethic of care is this or that but, in applying the elements of ethics and caring either to real situations or to issues, it will be evident that this is done from within an ethic of care, and at every juncture this will be indicated. (See also Ch. 1, 'Caring and ethics in nursing' by Stan van Hooft in the companion volume to this book, *Approaches to Ethics: Nursing Beyond Boundaries* (2003).) First, however, it is useful to consider some specific aspects of care and caring.

CARING

In a small book simply entitled *On Caring*, Milton Mayeroff (1972) lists eight 'major ingredients' as necessary for caring. He describes these specifically in the context of a parent caring for a child, a teacher for a pupil, a psychotherapist for a patient, or a husband for his wife. Nurses are rarely in such a close or extended relationship with patients, but Mayeroff's concern is 'to show that there is a common pattern of helping the other grow' (p. 1), which is very much what nurses do. In Virginia Henderson's (1964) famous words, nurses 'assist the individual, sick or well, in the performance of those activities contributing to health or its recovery (or to a peaceful death) that he would perform unaided if he had the necessary strength, will or knowledge' (p. 63).

Nurses do not necessarily help people to 'grow up', but they certainly help them to grow in understanding of their illness and how to cope with it. For many people, that is one of the biggest undertakings in their life.

Knowledge

In caring we need to know many things: who the other is, what that person's needs are, and what helps the other. We also need to know ourselves, and our strengths and limitations. We know some things explicitly and others implicitly. 'One important reason, perhaps, for our failure to realize how much knowing there is in caring is our habit sometimes of restricting knowledge arbitrarily to what can be verbalized' (Mayeroff 1972, p. 10). Knowledge is conveyed both verbally and non-verbally.

Patricia Munhall (1993) described cogently that nurses also need to learn how to 'unknow' in order to be authentically present for patients. This is not easy. However, unknowing—a kind of receptivity or humility—is essential if we want to hear the other person and learn what this person is and is about.

Alternating rhythms

We move between past experience and the present situation, between narrow and wide frameworks, between attention to detail and attention to the whole. We learn from the past and act now; we are active at one moment and inactive at another. Both parts are necessary; both are part of caring. There is a rhythm that includes all aspects, and also moves and alternates between them.

Patience

We do not wait passively for something to happen, we give it our full attention. However, like an idea, or the growth of a child, the growth of a person into full potential may take time. When we care, we have patience with people and proceed at their pace. That can be frustrating, but it is vital if real caring is to take place.

Honesty

This is a positive, often active, confrontation between ourselves and the other. We need to see the other as that person is, not as we would like that individual to be. It is more than simply not telling a lie. It is a kind of transparency and openness that respects the other.

Trust

Trust involves an appreciation of the other, of that person's independent existence. When we care too much, when we 'overprotect' the other, then we are not mutually trusting. Trusting also means that we have confidence in our ability to help. We must trust ourselves and our instincts. We must also trust the other, and this includes an element of risk, of letting go, of leaping into the unknown.

Humility

When we are open to each person and situation, then each relationship is unique. We cannot simply do what we did in the last case; we have to learn all the time. This learning means constant restarting, or 'unknowing'. Humility sees others as existing for themselves, not as means of self-fulfilment. Caring teaches us our true limitations and strengths. We accept both with humility.

Hope

Hope is not wishful thinking, but an expression of the fullness of the present, a present alive with a sense of the possible. Sometimes we have great hopes that a patient will achieve something, but such hopes may impoverish the present by making it largely a postponement for a 'more real' future. It is the moment itself that matters and that has the seeds for 'more'. The seeds need attention now. The process of caring is possible only because hope is always present.

Courage

In caring and in growing, we go into the unknown. Courage makes risk-taking possible. Yet courage is not blind. It is informed by knowledge of the past and by trust in our own and the other's ability to grow.

Caring can only be experienced, and the quality of that experience is what matters. These 'ingredients' help to shape the quality of caring in general.

THE 'FIVE Cs' OF CARING

The Canadian nurse-philosopher M Simone Roach (1992) has also established a set of aspects of caring. These are related particularly to nursing, but grow out of her general statement that 'Caring is the human mode of being' (p. ix). Mayeroff (1972) says similarly that, in 'caring, a man lives the meaning of his own life' (p. 2). Care is the basic element of being a person. When we do not care, we lose our 'being', and caring is the way back into 'being'.

The old division was that doctors cure and nurses care. Yet, care is basic and a precondition of cure, and, as a doctor once said, caring was done long before curing was done (Nouwen et al 1982).

Caring embodies certain qualities and specific characteristics. Roach (1992) has noted that these all start with the letter 'C': compassion, competence, confidence, conscience and commitment.

Compassion

Compassion may be defined as a way of living born out of an awareness of one's relationship to all living creatures (Roach 1992 p. 58).

Although this is not quite the correct translation of the word, something done with compassion is something done 'with passion'. Compassion has come to attention in recent years in various settings, not least of which is the influence of Buddhism, where compassion 'is understood mainly in terms of empathy – our ability to enter into and, to some extent, share others' suffering.' This compassion is 'unconditional, undifferentiated and universal in scope. A feeling of intimacy towards all other sentient beings, including those who would harm us, is generated' (Dalai Lama 1999, pp. 131–132). Compassion is often the response of a gut feeling to a situation of great need or 'passion'. It is a specific act in response to a specific need. Nouwen and co-authors (1982) wrote that:

Compassion asks us to go where it hurts, to enter into places of pain, to share in brokenness, fear, confusion and anguish. Compassion challenges us to cry out with those in misery, mourn with those who are lonely, to weep with those in tears. Compassion requires us to be weak with the weak, vulnerable with the vulnerable, and powerless with the powerless. Compassion means full immersion in the condition of being human (p. 4).

Compassion is more than simple kindness. It is also more than caring; we can care without having compassion. Compassion is something both decisive and incisive:

The wounded surgeon plies the steel
that questions the distempered part;
Beneath the bleeding hands we feel
the sharp compassion of the healer's art
Resolving the enigma of the fever chart (Eliot 1944, p. 29).

There is in this poem the implication that compassion comes only after an experience of being wounded oneself. When we have been 'bleeding' ourselves, and have experienced compassion towards us, then we can - out of that experience - in turn be healers. Compassion is something that we know only by experience. We cannot learn how to have or apply it. We cannot study it; no programme in sensitivity will give it to us. We can be compassionate only because compassion has been shown towards us.

Anthony Tuckett (1999) writes similarly that:

[Nurses] care when they are present with another with a closeness that evokes compassion. Hence, the caring nurse is focused on 'the other' so that 'the other's' welfare is paramount. This 'other regardingness' to which the caring nurse gives precedence means becoming emotionally involved. ... Nurses ought to respond in a caring way that is reasonable rather than exact (p. 387).

Larry Churchill (1977) believes that, in nursing:

Compassion is the groundwork, competence the superstructure. Usually in thinking of health professionals, we reverse this; we try to train a competent professional, and tack on compassion as a finishing touch icing on the cake, a highly desirable frill. To me this bespeaks a root poverty of our ability to really see what health professionals do, and how deeply they generally affect the lives of those they serve (p. 873).

Nouwen and co-authors (1982) believe that today competition, not compassion, is our main motivation in life. We judge people by what they do, their job, profession or rank, not by who they are. Being compassionate, however, is first of all acknowledging the other as a person, and that means going beyond dividing lines, differences and distinctions, even going against competitiveness. Nouwen and his co-authors' (1982) book, *Compassion*, is based on the life of a doctor in Paraguay whose son was tortured to death. Through this the father had come to see compassion also as a political force by 'defending the weak and indignantly accusing those who violate their humanity; joining with the oppressed in their struggle for justice; pleading for help with all possible means, from any person who has ears to hear and eyes to see' (p. 141).

Nurses are often in similar positions. By being advocates, taking professional decisions, challenging management decisions, questioning treatments on the grounds of conscience or values, nurses defend the weak and stand up with them against violations against humanity. For this to be compassion and not just self-interest, we need to know from where this attribute comes, and what are its aims.

Compassion is a complex aspect of caring. It demands above all a knowledge of one's self and one's values. To some extent, when we do not know ourselves, we are hurting others and making them into victims, or creating tensions that then require others to be compassionate to those we have hurt, however unconsciously.

Compassion is more specific than caring. Compassion questions, brings to closure, and defends others. Caring calls forth caring; compassion is there when it hurts. Caring can be professional, but compassion has to be experienced. Caring can be learnt, but compassion comes out of the experience of having been hurt and having been shown compassion. We do not respond with compassion out of a sense of duty, but out of a sense of solidarity.

Competence

Competence is a state of having the knowledge, judgement, skills, energy, experience and motivation required to respond adequately to the demands of one's professional responsibilities (Roach 1992, p. 61).

Competence distinguishes the expert from the novice. It is that which every nurse longs for and works towards during basic and post-basic education and training.

Competence has also become a political issue in recent years. Clause 6 of the Nursing and Midwifery Council (NMC) *Code of Professional Conduct* (2002) (see Ch. 5) is devoted to the maintenance of professional knowledge, and the competence of registered nurses and midwives. The NMC, as the United Kingdom Central Council before it, is concerned that nursing practice is 'lawful, safe and effective' (Cl. 6.2), rather than the other way round. The Code lays a specific duty on a practitioner to seek help if any part of practice required is beyond the person's level of competence (Cl. 6.3). This is reasonable, but the pressure is often intense (due mainly to shortage of staff) to go beyond the limit. In this sense, competence has become an issue of power and manipulation.

Roach warns that care will be diminished if competence becomes manipulation. Perhaps too many nurses have suffered from the small amounts of power that those working in a strict hierarchy have, and have been at the receiving end of personal insults, put-downs and being ignored (see Ch. 9). The weightier aspects of power that can easily be abused are not considered here, but only acknowledged.

Caring *does* demand competence, but competence with a human face. Care has to be appropriate, adequate, and practised with respect, considering the needs of those who are the recipients. In this way competence is very close to compassion; one tempers the other and one enhances the other by emphasising that opposites need each other. Competence also gives nurses the sense of achievement and confidence to practice. However, particularly in areas such as nursing and midwifery, levels of competence shift constantly, and it is right that a public body regulates competence and lays on its practitioners the duty to keep their knowledge and skills updated throughout their working life (Nursing and Midwifery Council 2002, Cl. 6.1).

Confidence

Confidence is defined as the quality that fosters trusting relationships (Roach 1992, p. 62).

Most nurses would agree that at the basis of caring lies a trusting relationship. Without that the whole ethos of caring is lost.

Confidence is reciprocal; both parties in a relationship need to trust each other. When one of the parties is in a professional position, then the other certainly needs to be sure that the professional can be trusted. This will depend largely on the degree of honesty (see Ch. 4) between them.

There is evident today a general erosion of confidence in most major institutions. People are wary of claims made by governments, managements of all kinds, advertising and the media. Health care has suffered a good deal also, not least because of individuals such as Dr Harold Shipman, and the Bristol heart surgery and Alder Hey Children's Hospital organ retention affairs. Nurses have not escaped, and some, like Beverley Allitt, have done a lot of damage to the profession. In an effort to counter this, codes of practice have been updated and professional bodies have been overhauled. Once damage has been done, it is very difficult to regain confidence. Individuals have to work much harder to be, and be seen to be, 'squeaky clean'.

If caring is to remain the unique feature of nursing, then confidence plays a large part. Genuine caring fosters confidence without coercion; it communicates truth without violence; it creates relationships that are not paternalistic or grounded on fear or powerlessness, but are based on sharing and mutual respect.

Conscience

The word 'conscience' can be defined as a state of moral awareness; a compass directing one's behaviour according to the moral fitness of things (Roach 1992, p. 63).

Conscience is at the basis of ethical behaviour. Roach (1992) has a number of aphorism-like statements that help to explain this concept.

Conscience is an intentional response, deliberate, meaningful and rational.
Conscience is the caring person attuned to the moral nature of things.
Conscience is the call of care and manifests itself as care.
Professional caring is reflected in a mature conscience (p. 64).

Conscience, as the faculty within, is learned from early childhood onwards, and grows and develops. Parents and teachers instil a sense of right and wrong, and this eventually forms the value basis on which judgements and decisions are made. Conscience is sometimes equated with 'feeling': feeling bad about doing something. The feeling may very well be the indicator that something fundamental is at stake. 'Claims of conscience commit the individual person to act morally' (Johnstone 1994, p. 451).

The claim to conscience is so strong that most people would not go against it, or force anybody to go against their conscience. Conscience is a loyalty to oneself that should be respected in ourselves and in others as an innate right, and as a duty in responding to something greater than ourselves. When conscience is allowed to be dulled or rationalised, it can result in behaviour that may be less than admirable or excellent.

Because caring is essentially vulnerable, conscience is the element that directs a person into the right behaviour: the good, the creative and compassionate way of relating. It is perhaps the most spiritual of the Five Cs, and the one that demands the most constant attention in the ways described above by Mayeroff (1972), through knowledge, humility and courage.

Commitment

Commitment is: *'a complex affective response characterized by a convergence between one's desires and one's obligations, and by a deliberate choice to act in accordance with them'* (Roach 1992, p. 65).

If the Five Cs were along a line, commitment would come last. Commitment somehow confirms the other Cs. Similarly, the other attributes all have to be present for commitment to be viable.

The idea of commitment has also been described as devotion (Mayeroff 1972, p. 5). Alastair Campbell (1984a) writes that 'consistent professional care is a form of love which entails a personal commitment by the person offering care' (p. 6). In a chapter on commitment, Stan van Hooft (1995) writes that commitment 'is a stance towards the world or towards others on the part of an individual or group which defines what is important or imperative for the individual or group' (p. 13).

Commitment then, is that certain 'stickability' that gets a person involved with another person, or a cause or a task, without sentimentality or sense of burden. Commitment is a response to a need or call that is somehow natural because caring is the human mode of being. Once the commitment is made—formally or informally, consciously at the time or only in retrospect—then it lasts for the duration of the relationship with the person, cause or action, and it steers the relationship positively.

This aspect of care is particularly evident in community nursing, where care is often given over many weeks or months, or even years. Carers who look after elderly or disabled relatives or neighbours for years, without any help or remuneration, show commitment to a very high degree.

THE CARE-GIVER

Caring is something practical, something done to some*one* by some*one*. We therefore need to look at the persons who give and receive care. Books about nursing sometimes concentrate on the patient and see the nurse only as the dispenser of care. Yet, as the

Five Cs show, care-givers have to have a great deal of self-knowledge, self-understanding and self-assertiveness. Therefore, to start with the nurse here seems logical.

A great deal has been written about self-awareness and how to achieve it, often in the psychological literature (e.g. Nelson-Jones 1982, Tschudin 1991, Tschudin with Schober 1998). The emphasis here is not so much on the act of self-awareness, as on what this eventually implies.

Caring involves for the care-giver first of all a 'feeling' with the other (Noddings 1984). This is perhaps best captured in the word 'empathy', which basically means 'suffering-in'. Suffering is subjective; it is a 'feeling'. To understand suffering, a person has to be 'in'. It is not a question of being in the sufferer's shoes, or even: 'How would I feel in that position?' It is a question of understanding the sufferer in that person's own position. It is not a question of projecting oneself into the other; it is a question of *receiving* the other into oneself. This may sound contrary to much that has been written about caring. On deeper reflection, however, it can be seen that caring based on relationship can only be *received* caring. One cares for the other; one receives the other.

The philosopher Martin Buber (1937) has expressed the basic relationships that exist in terms of 'I and It', and 'I and Thou'. I and It is the world of history, of objects and of the past. It is the world of things, and of experience, perceiving, imagining, wanting, sensing and thinking. The world of I and Thou is the world of relation: 'When *Thou* is spoken, the speaker has no *thing*; he has indeed nothing. But he takes his stand in relation' (p. 17).

Buber describes how the word-set I–It appears as ego; that is, the I becomes conscious of itself, and of experience and use. In the word-set I–Thou, the I speaks as a person. Egos set themselves apart, but persons enter into relation with other persons. The purpose of relating is relating. In doing so, we touch a Thou; something greater is given. As soon as there is a relation, there is something greater. Buber's notion of relating is not necessarily possible in nursing because it describes a deep spiritual engagement with the other. However, this kind of relationship cannot be ruled out and, in common with many other writers on caring, it is given as an example of the kind of relationship that is possible and even desirable in certain circumstances.

This 'given' described by Buber is known by all nurses. It is not the things given by the carer (the skills, the long hours, the tiredness, the unpleasant tasks) that matter. These are only what can be measured. What is received——what the patients give to nurses: the appreciation of a relative, the smile of a sick child, knowing that we have 'been there' when it mattered—these are the reasons why nursing is so unique. Which nurses have not been told 'I wanted to die—you don't know what you have done for me' (Allen 1992) and in truth *not* knowing what it was they did that made a person want to live.

This sort of caring and being with another person is what caring really means and what nurses invariably say they want to do most. The technical, scientific and administrative elements of care are its bedrock, but they cannot give that sense of satisfaction that comes from knowing that we have made a difference in a person's life. This is not simply sentimentality. Anyone who has ever been at the receiving end of care knows only too well just how important personal contact is when one is vulnerable. Care-givers have a duty to respect other people, and not only to listen to them but also to hear them. When care-giving becomes friendship and perhaps support, this needs to be acknowledged and possibly nurtured. If nurses knew that support will be available, they may be more ready to enter into either long-term or significant relationships (Baillie 1996).

Caring *is* about process, and science, and detachment. It is also about feeling (in-suffering) and about protecting and communicating. It is a kind of masculine approach that sees things in a linear way, and a feminine approach that sees things in a circular or spiral way. It is about giving and receiving. In order that the humanity of the persons concerned is not only maintained but enhanced, both masculine and feminine sides have to have their place in the scheme of things.

It is right that feminists have made us aware of the supremacy of caring, and also of the dangers of caring. Our motivations for caring are crucial. It has been argued that people who become nurses may have been hurt or neglected as a child and that (unconsciously) they seek to be 'healed' in the places where the sick are healed (i.e. hospitals), and that the best way to ensure this healing is by becoming a nurse (Tschudin 1997). The problem is that neither a hospital nor the nursing profession is very kind to such motivations and, rather than finding healing, nurses end up hurt and disillusioned. It may not be on entering nursing school that we are aware of our deep motives, but they have a way of escaping despite ourselves. How then do nurses care for people who pose immediate challenges?

- How does a nurse care for a patient on dialysis who is also an alcoholic?
- How does a nurse care for a 'lifer' who is transferred to a hospital for intensive chemotherapy?
- How does a nurse care for an elderly woman in her own home who is abusive and uncooperative, but will allow no one near her except the nurse?

Care can be care only when it is reciprocal. More than that, care has to be given to a person and received by a person. When the carer cannot give care in the way that individual would like to, the person is diminished. Equally, when the cared-for is not received by the carer as a person, the carer is diminished in that individual's humanity. For care to be genuine, both people in the relationship have to be received. The main element of such receiving is listening.

Any care given may be competent but, if compassion, confidence or commitment are lacking, it is hollow care. This is where the carer's capacity for self-awareness and self-assessment is crucial. This is the work of conscience. Stepping back and examining what is happening, and perhaps taking stock of positions that may need to change, is what receiving the other through listening is about.

Such self-searching is not easy. It can quickly become an inward-looking exercise that simply leads to more retrenched positions and one-sided views. The carer too needs care, and needs to be heard. Caring can be given only by a person who has also been heard. The person who cares for another who is over-demanding or unresponsive needs to be heard by someone else. Only thus is the circle of care closed; or, rather, it is a spiral that allows a person not just to go round and round, but up and down, seeing the problem from different levels.

Real caring demands a human person's fullest capacity to respond to the needs of another person, and in doing that there are sometimes situations that demand more than the usual, or catch us at unprepared moments or at a time of personal struggle. These times and moments are challenges. To brush them aside, leaving our feelings at the door, is unrealistic and dehumanising. We become truly human and truly caring only through challenge, suffering and suffering-in. That has to be learned, sustained and cared-for.

THE CARE-RECEIVER

In nursing we tend to think of the one who receives care as a patient. This basically implies someone who is static, ill and receptive. The terms 'client' or 'customer' are also being used increasingly. This gives an emphasis of someone who shops for a particular article and pays for it. Neither of these terms are really satisfactory. Nurses are also in close professional touch with the families and friends of those cared for, and with colleagues and indeed all those who make up the caring team. By using the term care-receiver the problem is not made easier, but it is intended to include all those with whom nurses are professionally in touch.

Even though it is declining, our culture still stresses giving to and pleasing others: 'There is more happiness in giving than in receiving.' Although we can and do teach how to give care, we usually do not teach how to receive; we just expect that people know how to do it when they are in a situation where they cannot avoid it. This may actually be the wrong way round. Only when we know how to receive can we also give.

It can be argued that everyone knows how to receive because children receive their parents' care. This cannot simply be taken for granted. Most adults suffer in life from one aspect or another of the care given or withheld, or given wrongly, by their parents. When they are then ill, or at some particular stage in life when they receive care, they may not know how to accept it. Equally, with the fragmentation of family life in society, some people, particularly those who are elderly, have become so independent that they reject any care that is well-meaning enough but may be seen by them as an intrusion.

Other people may do just the opposite and squeeze every ounce of care out of the system and the people around them.

These are the extremes at both ends of the spectrum but, so that the norm can be seen more clearly, they have to be acknowledged. In these instances, what is going on is not so much care-giving and receiving, but ego-tripping. The care-receiver is not able any more to say Thou to another, hence this person's I becomes isolated. Care in this instance, if solution orientated, entirely misses the point, because it does not address the person.

The care that is person orientated is very different. We have all been in situations when we felt that we were the only person in the whole world who mattered to someone. It was not just a giving and a receiving of something, but a being together of two people. This implies that both were heard, and that hearing enhanced their humanity. It is out of such experiences that giving grows and becomes the sort of giving that selflessly enhances another.

This sort of giving should be the experience of the care-receiver. The cared-for person is the only one who matters at that moment. That person 'fills the firmament', as Noddings (1984, p. 74) puts it. The care-giver is engrossed in the other. This presupposes an acceptance of the care-receiver that is non-judgemental.

When we are caring for a prisoner, or a cantankerous woman, we are judging them by a label given for a purpose. We have to judge others in order to maintain our value system; but they also force us to question that value system. One person was particularly upset when her husband was described as being 'away with the fairies' simply because he could not speak after a stroke. She remembers this with pain, but she was also much encouraged when another nurse asked her what her husband was like before he had the stroke (Anonymous 2001c).

In order to meet the person we need to go beyond the appearance, the label, the misdeed, and particularly beyond our own fears and hang-ups; these are the things that block real care-giving and receiving more than the weightier matters of moral behaviour.

In Buber's term, the other person is or becomes Thou. When we are really able to address a person as Thou then we are with that person in a relationship that is not one-sided. We do not become over-involved in or absorbed by the other. When we truly say Thou to someone, we see that person as that person is: individual, worthy of care and full of potential. It is so often in the paradox that we see the real situation; when I say Thou truly, then I become truly I. In acknowledging the other as a person in that individual's own right by saying Thou, I receive myself, because I have cared; but I cannot give of myself in order to receive. I give in order to give, and in doing that I receive.

THE CARING RELATIONSHIP

The caring relationship is the basis of an ethic of caring. How and what that relationship is and comprises is therefore of particular importance.

Using the images of masculine and feminine, the masculine aspect of being human tends to isolation, to independence and to detachment. These are necessary elements of living and functioning, and are not debated here. The feminine aspect of being human is more at home with 'receptivity, relatedness and responsiveness' (Noddings 1984, p. 2). These aspects are specifically needed for a caring relationship and are highlighted here but dealt with more specifically in the next chapter.

The caring done in nursing comes out of the sense of relating because something or someone has been received. This is in contrast to what much recent western philosophy has advocated (including bioethics), that the starting point of ethics is freedom, or autonomy. These theories hold that an individual is an autonomous agent who can and must be free to decide. This presupposes an aloneness and an emptiness at the heart of existence within which moral decisions must be made. Noddings (1984, p. 6) argues that this position leads to anguish directed at the responsibility that this aloneness and freedom demand. This is evident in the now mainly discarded stance of a (male) doctor who believes that a decision concerning a patient is his and his alone (it usually was a man). Women, on the other hand, who are experiencing relatedness, experience with that not anguish, but joy. This is a joy of being with, of belonging and of receiving.

By making this point, the masculine anguish is not denigrated, but rather highlights what has perhaps been obvious to many nurses: in caring we are fulfilled; when simply fighting a dilemma, we are alienated. This is equally true for men and women. In psychological terms a person is truly integrated when a man accepts the feminine aspects in himself and a woman accepts the masculine aspects in herself. In a caring relationship, therefore, both masculine and feminine aspects play a part: the masculine capacity to separateness is as important as the feminine capacity for inclusion. This is a clear aspect of empathy. Empathy needs the 'feeling-in' aspect to begin with, and also the 'letting-go' or standing back later. In stressing the feminine aspects here, legitimacy is given to those facets of care that are still often devalued and overlooked in models and theories that emphasise strictly linear approaches, or models that are too clinical and symptom orientated rather than inclusive and holistic.

The Five Cs of caring—compassion, competence, confidence, conscience and commitment—are able to function only within a relationship. A person on a desert island is certainly able to exercise these aspects towards self, and to animals, plants and ideas. However, this is limited because, although plants and animals give us something, they do not reciprocate any feelings, and such a person is seriously at risk of mental instability.

Caring rests on feelings, and on the memories and hopes that they produce. Where helping and caring are involved, the feelings tend to relate to suffering, taking suffering in the widest sense. When caring is given by one human being to another human being, and a relationship is created whereby some helping played a part (whatever that helping was), then the main feeling that both are left with is joy. We are often too inhibited to call it joy; but feeling good, being cheerful, walking tall, job satisfaction, glowing with pride, and also the deep inner affirmation of having helped someone and knowing it, are all aspects of joy.

A true relationship is not established on any rules. Caring has to be done within certain parameters and standards, usually laid down by an employing authority, the regulatory body of the professional, the status of the carer, and the position of the care-receiver. These limits and rules must be acknowledged, but also set aside when necessary, for a relationship to happen.

The relationship between nurses and those they care for is often very unequal: one is sick, one is healthy; one is ignorant, one is knowledgeable; one is receiving, one is giving; one is in need, the other fulfils the need. These divisions and boundaries are, however, disappearing as patients and clients are better informed and less passive about health care. The relationship therefore becomes much more one of equals, but this is not always easy for professionals who have studied for a long time to gain expertise.

The hallmark of professionals is that they share their expert knowledge with their client. Professionals put their advantage at the disposal of the client. (In contrast, non-professional workers do what they are asked to do.) These issues have far-reaching ethical implications, in particular with regard to informed consent (see Ch. 9). Yet this stance still implies that one is superior, another inferior.

Campbell (1984a) describes 'companionship' as the defining mark of the nurse–patient relationship. The care-giver is a companion (the literal translation of the word means 'with-bread', an evocative symbol) 'who shares freely, but does not impose, allowing others to make their journey' (p. 49). The companion softens the hardness of the journey the patient is on, whether this is recovery or death. Companionship is less than friendship, but it is still willing to share risks. However, the commitment of companionship is limited, and parting is an essential element in companionship. This model of relationship is less all-encompassing than Buber's I–Thou relationship and has more of a sense of a practical empathy about it.

The people for whom nurses care in particular are all sick or injured, in body, mind or spirit. Suffering is therefore the starting point. The goal for all is a restoration to health or recovery (or a peaceful death). It is greater wholeness that we all strive for, nurses and patients, and their families and friends. In this we are one; in this we are not different. With these given things therefore, the relationship between care-givers and care-receivers is essentially directed already. A caring relationship is necessary if getting well is seen not just as a process, like a necessary evil time that one has to pass through, but is to be a creative time for which some meaning is at least possible if not essential. Nurses who can help patients or clients to see this time of healing as a time of wider perspectives, of challenges and springboards to greater integrity and creativity, are nurses who are truly in touch with their own creativity. Creativity never happens alone. Anything creative happens within relationships, not just between humans, but also in relationships with ideas and objects. When the care-giver is in touch with this and can call this creativity forth in the other, then there is relating and there is joy; in a sense then, the I is no more I, and the Thou is no more Thou, but there is a 'We'.

Is the care-receiver wanting to be in touch with such elements? Creativity is the most fundamental instinct of being human. This is not just procreation, but a creativity that is fruitful even when it is not fertile. It is a creativity that stems from a deep sense of needing to say Thou to something greater than ourselves, and therefore tends towards that Thou where alone it finds fulfilment. Health, or restoration to health, is part of this creativity, as is eventually a relinquishing of life so that the greater can come. Thus the care-receiver is in touch with all this, even if not always consciously.

An example of such caring, and as a bridge from this to the next chapter, the following story speaks for itself:

A female nurse in her fifties comes on duty one morning and is asked to care for two men who have both had heart attacks. One of them had suffered only a minor attack. She helps him to get out of bed and he leaves the room. The other, a man approximately her own age, had suffered a worse attack and is very depressed and lies immobile in his bed. The stubble of his beard is getting long and his look is empty. The nurse goes about her business in the room for a while before she walks up to the bed and says: 'Tell you what, I'm very good at shaving men in the old-fashioned way with a brush and razor. I'd like to shave your face.' The man does not reply, nor does he seem to object. She prepares the brush and razor, soap and hot water. With care she soaps his face and shaves him. She dries his face after shaving and applies cream to moisturize the skin. Then she suggests that she should wash his hands. She leaves each of his hands in a bowl with soap and warm water for some minutes before drying them and applying moisturizer. Finding the result to her satisfaction, she looks at the patient, who is still immobile. She leaves him to rest but goes about her business on the ward for as long as she is on duty. The following day she works at the intensive care unit and does not meet her patient again. However, four weeks later she runs into him in town. He recognizes her and comes up to her. 'I think you saved my life the day you shaved me and washed my hands', he says. 'You made me feel that life was worth living after all' (Lindseth 2001, p. 392).

2

Relationship issues

MODELS OF RELATIONSHIPS

It is possible to see ethics in terms of ideals to be pursued. A caring relationship may therefore be an 'ideal' relationship. This does not diminish it; on the contrary, it is an ideal to strive for, and like a light leading the way.

In order to highlight the characteristics of an ethical relationship it is useful to look at the different ways in which relationships can be described.

Robert Veatch (1972) has outlined four types of relationships that doctors have with patients: priestly, engineering, contractual and collegial models. These also apply to nurses, particularly with the increase of primary nursing.

The priestly model

The priestly model is paternalistic. In this type of relationship the patient is passive, and the doctor or nurse 'plays God'. Any decision, particularly of an ethical nature, is the privilege or burden of the doctor, acting totally alone. The patient's values are not considered and not asked for. This model of a relationship is essentially unethical because the patient's consent in matters that affect that person's life is not requested. The exceptions are 'incompetent' patients: those who are unconscious, those who are severely mentally handicapped or ill, and children below the age of consent.

The engineering model

In the engineering model the health-care provider is seen to be the 'scientist'. Patients are given all the facts, so that they can then make their own choice. Health professionals become like plumbers, cleaning out drains, as they service the wishes of patients. This model of relationships is basically unsatisfactory because neither the values nor the emotions of either patient or carer are taken into account, but only the bare facts.

The contractual model

The contractual model is very different. In this relationship the patient's values are explored and discussed. The nurse (or doctor) is of vital importance as a 'collaborator' on decisions to be taken.

This model is most closely allied to the concept of caring. It is also essentially the model advocated by the nursing process. It shows a respect for the person, and is built on a relationship of sharing, enhancing each other and respecting each other's needs and values.

The collegial model

The collegial model is highly idealistic. Both patient and nurse share mutual goals and act as 'pals'. Decisions are reached by consensus. However, even Veatch (1972) agrees that this model is rather impractical.

THE 'NEW NURSING'

The term 'new nursing' was coined by Jane Salvage (1990) to describe an internal reform movement, which she believes dates back to the early 1970s and is basically an ideology of partnership. The background to this movement can be sketched by a few broad outlines.

Without doubt, the introduction of the nursing process had started a revolution in nursing. The task-orientated approach gave way to the patient-orientated approach. This was further highlighted when nursing models came on to the scene. These new ways of working demanded that nurses ask some fundamental questions about care and the relationships between themselves and patients, and between themselves and doctors. It was not so much a question any more of what is a nurse, or what nurses do, but: What is nursing? The answers have to do with 'receptivity, relatedness and responsiveness' (Noddings 1984, p. 2), pointing to values, to meaning and to community. In practical terms, this is characterised by assertiveness among nurses and a move away from the disease-orientated medical model to a holistic model of care.

Movements towards equality between the sexes in pay, status, education and job opportunities have fostered an assertiveness that was unknown to many people. Nurses have often been portrayed as angels, handmaids, sex symbols or domineering matrons; they have also colluded with these images. As assertiveness grows in strength, these stereotypes lose their hold. Nurses no longer have to project an image in order to be accepted or taken seriously. Yet assertiveness does not come easily after a long time of submissive 'second fiddle' status.

With some of these influences in the background, Salvage (1990) believes that two opposing ideologies advocate partnership: those who draw on the ideals of humanistic psychology and the one-to-one relationship; and those who defend the market forces and competitive strategies. Basically, both sides are about power relations. When nurses see themselves as partners, however, the need for power and defence of power is diminished drastically.

The new nursing is practised as such mainly in nursing development units in the UK. In these units, nurses are in charge rather than doctors and thus the traditional hierarchy is not needed; a primary nurse enters a partnership with the patient and so there is more consistent care.

Salvage (1990) makes the point that many patients judge the quality of nursing by its 'emotional style'. She is not alone in this; the many care studies published in the nursing press week by week put increasing emphasis on this aspect of care. Patients neither expect nor want a quasi-psychotherapeutic relationship with the nurse, but look for 'warmth, kindness and sensitivity' (p. 44) when delivering care and treatments. The partnership is thus based on the human need to be relieved from pain and discomfort. The way in which this is done is significant. 'Any nurse can stick a needle or an enema into anything human, and for that matter into beings which are not human. But not all nurses can supply optimum care to all patients' (Jourard 1971, pp. 202–203).

The idea of partnership with the patient or client stems from the sense of 'being in this together', a sense of a common destiny. The individual (I) who becomes or is more assertive does not care for any self-gain. The individual cares for another (Thou). Real care is always other-directed. Real care is also more than just helping to heal a broken limb by keeping the traction functioning. Real care is helping the person to adjust to the broken limb and then to adjust to life in that new situation, finally to integrate the whole event into the wider context of health and illness. Some patients do this with ease and seemingly without thinking about it; others need help, particularly if the illness is a serious one or threatens the person's livelihood. This is where the caring role of nurses is such a significant one. Their competence and experience, their compassion and commitment, is vital—although often not demonstrative—in helping clients and patients to make sense of their illness and limitations. Nurses are more than just the critical link with the outside world in a hospital; they are also often the link for patients between their external situation and their internal experience.

Sadly, Salvage (1990) concludes that not many nurses either do, or are inclined to, care in a partnership way. The patient-centred care is eroded by 'staff shortages, lack of time, the bureaucratic management system employed by most ward sisters, a mixture of organisational constraints and the emotional safety of routine work' (pp. 44–45).

Yet the increasing trend to more care in the community, and a slowly increasing understanding of patient-centred care, all contribute to more partnership. The model of disease orientation is giving way to a model of person orientation, where 'life' is seen as a whole. Disease, disability, old age and death are perceived less as 'bad' and enemies to be fought against, but are considered again as part of life and living. However, this is not without its problems. Increasing technology use is not necessarily increasing bliss. The more we know, the more we have to use this knowledge responsibly. Technology and knowledge can lead to increasing independence - but also to isolation. The new nursing, with its emphasis on partnership, is ideally placed consciously to balance this by the way it treats its 'partners' in 'receiving' them, relating to them and responding to them with care. In that way it is ideally a covenant relationship based on the gift of self.

3

Values and value statements

VALUES

We make value judgements and value statements all the time: what we wear; what, how and where we eat; how we travel; the friends we have; the place we live in. At every moment of our lives we reveal our values to ourselves and others.

Values are the personal aspects and foundations of social and ethical living. We probably feel most comfortable with people who hold similar values. Much of life is spent in adapting to circumstances we may not like and may not have chosen, but cannot escape. What we have to grapple with in life is often not what we would choose; thus we are urged on to find values where we never thought we would. Our moral and ethical decisions are based on values. We take our moral judgements seriously, so we also need to take our values seriously.

Values can be divided into three levels of expression: beliefs, attitudes and values themselves.

Beliefs

A belief is probably the most basic value and the one that changes least. A belief is a type of attitude that is based more on faith than fact. Anne Frank (1989) wrote in her diary that 'people are truly good at heart' (p. 330) three weeks before being captured by the Nazis and deported to a concentration camp, where she died.

A belief goes beyond the obvious, but at least it starts from the basis of some fact. One needs to have met some people who are good at heart in order to believe that all, or most, of them are good at heart.

Perhaps one of the main beliefs in nursing is that patients will get better with good care. Jane Salvage (2000) believes that there will be a breakthrough 'when policy-makers recognise that the knowledge and skills of caring have just as much impact on health and well-being as the knowledge and techniques appropriated by medicine' (p. 26).

Attitudes

An attitude is a disposition, or a settled behaviour. Attitudes are rather constant feelings, usually made up of different beliefs. They can be positive or negative.

Some of the attitudes particular to nursing are expressed in the way care is given. In describing the 'unique function of a nurse', Virginia Henderson (1964) says in the second part of her famous statement: 'The nurse is temporarily the consciousness of the unconscious, the love of life of the suicidal, the leg of the amputee, the eyes of the newly blind, a means of locomotion for the newborn, knowledge and confidence for the young mother, a voice for those too weak to speak, and so on.'

These are 'functions' that a nurse performs, but, without the attitudes based on the beliefs that they are valuable, no nurse could perform them. Moreover, Henderson believes that these functions are unique to nursing and that no other health workers could claim them or take them from nurses. Thus the attitudes with which they are performed are also unique to nursing.

Values

Values are less fixed, and more dynamic, than beliefs and attitudes because there is usually an element of motivation involved.

Louis Raths et al (1966) believe that people who are (or appear to be) flighty, apathetic, moody, rebellious, conforming and submissive, or phoney, may not have come to grips with their own values.

Viktor Frankl (1962) argued that the most important goal in life for each person is the search for meaning. A person finds meaning through values. Frankl writes as a person who spent most of the war years in concentration camps in Germany. He claims that those of his fellow inmates who saw meaning in their life did not succumb to the typhus infection that killed most of those who were not sent to the gas chambers. He speaks of three types of values: creative, experiential and attitudinal.

Creative values

Creative values are those that are discovered through what we do, particularly through helping others. Anyone can help someone to discover some values. Being a shop assistant is creative: a shop assistant may make customers aware that a certain colour suits them and this gives customers more confidence; another assistant may help someone to choose a tie for a special event and find just the right one. It is clear that nursing as a job will give more satisfaction than working on a conveyor belt. Helping people in any kind of way will always highlight some values; being of use to others strengthens the sense of self-worth, increases relationships and widens the emotional and intellectual horizon. Simply making a patient comfortable in bed gives a sense of achievement, but having relieved another person's distress means that a human need has been responded to, and that is what living is most deeply about.

Experiential values

Experiential values are those that are discovered through appreciation of people, events, and natural or artistic beauty.

Frankl points out that values cannot be created; they are discovered. We do not set out to make ourselves happy. We do something like going to a concert and the appreciation of the music makes us happy. A wonderful sunset or the sight of Niagara Falls can give one a sense of awe and wonder, and put one in touch with nature or with the infinite. These then become values and we may set out to experience them again. Before they were experienced for the first time, they may have been known about but not known to ourselves, nor would we know if we would or should choose them for ourselves.

The same is true of values about people. An honest person is known when meeting one, and that heightens the sense of the importance of honesty. The Queen, the Prime Minister, and Elvis Presley stand for certain ideals. We can accept their ideals or leave them, but the experience we have of the value of their ideals is important. It is not only the great and the good who inspire. Every nurse has been inspired by a dying child, a sick father, or an 'ordinary' patient who can lead nurses to discover values by being around them (i.e. by 'experiencing' these people simply for what they are and who they are).

Attitudinal values

Attitudinal values are those that are discovered through the way in which we react to unfortunate circumstances over which there is no control, such as our own and other people's suffering.

Frankl's main theory is that people need to have a meaning in life, and that their task is to search for this meaning. Thus illnesses, accidents and suffering of all kinds are triggers in that search, and sometimes the answer itself. Helen Oppenheimer (1995), whose basic premise is that 'people matter', and therefore what matters to people matters, says that 'mattering is more given than chosen' (p. 67). She explains that 'we have a lot of control over facts, but values are given to us' (p. 68). We can marry the person we choose, but we have no control over that person developing Alzheimer's disease. Yet, when this happens, we need to adjust to this and form our values about the partner's life, our own life, and how this situation fits into the wider context.

Anyone who has an accident or a serious illness will ask at some stage: Why? Why me? Why now? Why in this way? These questions, and the answers finally given to them, shape a person's life. When a person has discovered a meaning in life, then that person lives purposefully. The way in which we care for people who are ill will inevitably contribute to the discovery of meaning in their life and also in our own.

Values take on significance only when they are tested against someone or something. We may say that we value life, but it is probably only after an accident, illness, or a brush with death that we truly appreciate our own life.

Nursing values are constantly questioned. In the post-modern age, when 'anything goes' and there is little consensus on any issue, individuals defend their own stance. Such moral pluralism is possibly the reason why, as individuals and as a society, we are so aware of moral conflicts and dilemmas. We are constantly challenged to reinterpret and redefine: what nursing is or should be; what matters most in certain sectors of nursing; what nursing education is and is about; and what power in nursing is and is for. In Chapter 1 it was pointed out that self-awareness is at the basis of helping and listening. It is also at the basis of any study of values. Raths et al (1966) established a set of requirements that need to be present for a value to result. It is remarkable that their model has held so long and is still the basis of teaching on values.

It is necessary that the person:

1. Chooses freely.
2. Chooses from among alternatives.
3. Chooses after thoughtful consideration of the consequences of each alternative.
4. Prizes and cherishes them: one is happy with the choice made.
5. Affirms them: there is a willingness to affirm the choice publicly.
6. Acts upon the choices: they affect and give direction to actual living.
7. Repeats them: they become a pattern in one's life.

In summary, this means that choosing (1–3), prizing (4–5) and acting (6–7) make up the basis on which values rest.

This book suggests that caring is such a value. In choosing to become a nurse, a person chooses to care. Each person expresses this differently, but we can care either because we have to or because we want to. We may not like that we 'have to' care; that is, because it is part of the job and it is the only job available, and the mortgage has to be paid. How each person expresses care will not only be a personal moral or ethical choice but it will also be expressed in relationships with others, particularly in the way in which other people's values are respected.

Values are dynamic. Young people see objects and life in terms of right and wrong, black and white. Experience of living, mixing with people and discerning meaning will shape and change our values. The process of choosing, prizing and acting on is therefore a constantly repeating one. For some people, more and more things have value; others feel that, as they grow older, fewer and fewer values matter.

Values that are repeatedly threatened in ethics are those related to the value of life, such as human rights, dignity and respect. In the nursing setting, the values of care, health and health care also have a particular place.

VALUES OF CARING

Caring is a response to someone who matters, simply because the person is there. We respond to each person and situation differently but, in order to be truly human, we do need to respond. Not every person we meet is a friend, but each one is a person just like ourselves, and, as we matter, so they matter. People matter. When we consider someone as less worthy than ourselves, we diminish ourselves. Some people are cruel or not worthy of admiration, but morally they are no less persons than we are. Many people who have been tortured or imprisoned have kept themselves sane by seeing their keepers as sons of mothers who loved them and cared for them. Maybe the keepers cared for their mothers even while mistreating others. The elements of caring outlined in Chapter 1 matter here:

- Receptivity: the other is received as she, he or it is. In Manning's (1998) words (see Ch. 1), this constitutes moral attention and sympathetic understanding.
- Relatedness: receiving someone or something means to be in relation to her, him or it. Manning's relationship awareness fits here.
- Responsivity: receiving alone is not enough; receiving comes alive through responding. The person who responds calls forth a response in the other, and thus a relationship is created. Manning uses the terms 'accommodation' and 'response' with similar aims.

These values of relating need to be put alongside Roach's (1992) Five Cs as values of caring (see Ch. 1):

- Compassion
- Competence
- Confidence
- Conscience
- Commitment.

The following story may help to put abstract terms into the perspective of caring practice.

I remember in my nursing days having to care for a middle-aged man suffering from multiple sclerosis. F was rather overweight and much misunderstood. He had been moved from a medical to a geriatric ward because 'he was taking up too much of the nurses' time in an acute medical ward'. 'He's always moaning and complaining', I was told. I was on night duty on the senior citizens' ward when I first met F. In helping him to retire at night, I was constantly helping him to change his position. Every few minutes of the first half hour he would ask for his position to be changed, 'move my leg, move my arm, move my buttock,' he would say. It was always move this, move that, and he could be quite trying. However, I soon learned that if I took time to listen and hear F, and move him as and when he requested, it could mean spending 20–30 minutes with him.

Then finally, he would say, 'I'm fine now, thank you.' He would soon be asleep and would invariably sleep through the whole night. It was only when I could hear and feel his pain, his helplessness, through hearing and paying full attention to his requests, that I could respond to F ungrudgingly, giving him the possibility to go to sleep. This, I am sure, was because attention was being paid to him as a person rather than as a patient. It enabled him to feel that he was still valuable enough for someone to listen to him and to affirm him as a person who happened to be labelled a patient.

F taught me a great deal about having the patience not only to listen but, more importantly, how to hear. He also taught me how difficult it is to take time to listen to the pain of another who is constantly complaining that no one understands and that no one cares that he is full of pain. He needed me and my time to listen to the meaning of his pain. Naturally this is difficult when you have 20–30 other persons in the ward demanding the presence of your ears (B Kirkpatrick, personal communication, 1986).

The three 'Rs' of a caring ethic and the 'Five Cs' of Roach are all demonstrated in this story in different ways. Manning's comment (1998) that working with an ethic of care takes time is certainly demonstrated. However, the story also shows that there may be some self-interest in this too: the nurse who spent time with F did this only once during the night, whereas others might have spent much more time because of frequent calls from F to gain attention.

Some more general points about caring need to be made here in conjunction with this story and the values outlined above. Rogers (1961) listed some elements of helping relationships that he considered essential in counselling; these are also relevant here, where the relationship is the basis of caring.

Being

Before we can *do*, we need to *be*: be ourselves, one human person with another human person. This entails that we are trustworthy, honest, dependable. Rogers (1961) states that he used to think that being dependable and consistent meant keeping appointments, being always acceptant, and respecting confidence. He learned that *being* trustworthy or consistent does not demand a rigid consistency, but that he can be 'dependably real' (p. 50). This is much the same in nursing, particularly when a uniform can actually present a barrier to simply 'being' with another person.

Respect

We do not always like someone at first sight. In caring we respect a person first of all, and this may—sometimes surprisingly—lead to a mutual liking. Every nurse knows 'difficult patients' (like F) whose reputation has often gone before them. Getting to know the person rather than working on hearsay and assumptions is a very important starting point for caring. Our vulnerability expresses itself in very different ways, and fear and shame experienced by patients may express themselves in unsocial ways. Clearly, abusive behaviour should not be tolerated, but addressing the real person rather than the 'actor' may make all the difference.

Separateness and freedom

Even though we are caring, and deeply caring, we are not 'engulfed' by others, downcast by their depression, or frightened by their fear. Others need to be free to express themselves and be what they are even though we may not like some types of freedom. We need to remain separate persons. Perhaps the fear in nursing of 'getting involved' was the possible inability to step back from a relationship and not see oneself as separate, leaving neither party the necessary freedom. This is where true empathy matters.

Empathy

This is the ability to perceive the feelings of other persons, and the ability to communicate this to them (Kalisch 1971). When we can understand what goes on within ourselves, then we are better able to understand the world of the other. This gives us not only the ability but also the confidence to engage with the other person. Helping empathically and effectively means there is that 'separateness' that leaves us not burdened at the end of a helping episode, but rather with a sense of having grown as a person alongside the other.

Communication

Both our verbal and non-verbal communication should convey that we are 'for' this person. What we convey should correspond to what is relevant and encouraging. Communication is always the first and last need. We need to learn to respond to the other person's ways of communicating. This does not diminish us but in fact enables us to enlarge our own horizon.

Evaluation

Evaluation of a situation helps, but all too often we use and take evaluation personally. In caring we need to be clear and specific, as does the other person. When we help others to evaluate where they are in relation to where they have come from and where they want to go, then we care for and about them.

Becoming

All caring is so that the other can grow and become. The first element in this list is 'being', because this is what we start with in any situation. All helping is done so that the other person is in a better space or position at the end of the helping intervention. This infers that there needs to be a 'becoming'. With the elements here outlined we address the other person's potential. This demands a kind of optimism and a belief that what we are doing in any helping situation is that it is indeed helpful. The helping we are doing is not for ourselves, but for the other; we foster the other person. Yet in so doing we are helped ourselves; we 'become' more ourselves. Both parties are 'humanised' in this.

To be human is to care. Clearly, not all caring is always nice. Breakdown of relationships happens; feelings of anger, resentment, hate and destruction are often more powerful than their good opposites. Anger, fear, resentment and so on are legitimate and often helpful feelings. They are most destructive when they are expressed face to face. When the relationship can be of such a quality that these feelings can be addressed and explored, then not only does helping take place, but real healing and restoration are possible. This needs integrity from an individual helper (if a nurse is in such a position), but it also needs support from the organisation in which the individual works, and it needs a wider political commitment that helping and caring are necessary and are a 'good' that should be achieved.

VALUES OF HEALTH

The values of health are far from simple. In western medicine we have gone to great lengths to eradicate disease. The possibilities are in sight where we can choose not only the colour of the eyes of our offspring, but which diseases we avoid having, and, if we must have any diseases, to choose the time of life when to have them. Some of this still sounds rather Utopian, but we can be sure that somewhere some person is working at problems that are a few steps beyond what has not yet even penetrated the scientific world.

In his Reith Lectures, Jonathan Sacks (1990) made the point that without objective standards, we have no coherent language of ethics. We have largely lost a sense of obligations that constrain our choices, and duties that put limits on our desires. We are much more aware of autonomy, equality and rights as values that allow us as individuals to be whatever we choose. Sacks argued that we choose our own acts freely, but take it for granted that the consequences should be dealt with by the state. This has led to the situation where governments are expected to reduce child abuse, homelessness, sexually transmitted diseases and addiction, but cannot, or should not, disseminate a morality that could reduce these problems in the first place. In recent years it has become acceptable that smoking 'is bad for you' and no-smoking policies now apply in most hospitals. However, the same does not apply to obesity, which is a growing health problem in the western world. It is not politically correct to stop someone eating or not admit them to restaurants. There are no objective standards that are applicable to all people or all diseases, and therefore the language of one group of people offends that of another.

Care and cure are not value free. To think otherwise is 'malignant nonsense' according to Ivan Illich (1976, p. 56). In the years since Illich wrote, this has become even more evident. Most values concerning health are based on perceived need:

- What is the person's bodily or mental need? Who decides? Whose judgement is more valuable or acceptable: the doctor's or the patient's?
- What is the goal of the need? What state of health could be reached with care or treatment? Is it complete restoration or an acceptable state? Who is right?
- Which secondary effects of treatments are acceptable and which are not?
- Who has priority of treatment? For what reasons?
- How do we know when a frustrated disabled person needs help (and we give it), or when the person needs to learn to manage alone?

The perceived needs for, and in, health depend largely on the theories or concepts about health that a person holds. Per-Erik Liss and Lennart Nordenfelt (1990) point out that, in an analytical framework of health, statistical normality is the key concept, whereas a holistic theory views a whole person's function and activity. The values that arise from either of these approaches will colour the stance taken. The above statements look different, depending on which theory either party holds. The fact is that 'both the goal of need and the suitable treatment to reach the goal are things we choose' (Liss and Nordenfelt 1990, p. 113). Denise Rankin-Box (2000) believes that complementary therapies can be seen as either rational or irrational, but they are not unreasonable. What is 'reasonable' is very likely the measure for deciding on differing values in health care.

The choices of either party in a disagreement are based on values that have been accumulated with experience over the years. A person who had one 'bad' operation may put up with considerable discomfort before even contemplating having another. A doctor who has seen many patients with similar conditions will think it practically impossible for someone not to undergo a certain treatment despite 'a few' side-effects.

A very broad generalisation can perhaps be made about these views. A more masculine approach from a medical model of care is to see life and problems in terms of progression from A to B, in statistics, symptoms and prognoses. A more feminine view would be to see health in holistic terms of all-inclusive functioning and well-being, and of a nursing model of care. Women may be more likely to live with 'imperfection' in terms of health, and talk not of cure but of healing. Without the analytical approach, medicine would not be where it is today. Without the more holistic approach, medicine cannot survive. The debate goes on but, as it does so, it is widening into a public debate, and even a political debate. Nurses need to be aware of this and dare to take the stance that is most applicable to their situation, and to the well-being of their patients and clients.

VALUES OF HEALTH CARE

It is a truism that every aspect of health care is constantly changing. What applies today may not apply tomorrow. If the values governing caring all begin with the letter C, those of businesses and organisations tend to begin with the letter E: economy, efficiency and effectiveness.

Most of western society is committed to a capitalist system based on the idea of the market and trade. Goods should be freely available and customers have the choice of what to buy. This is also increasingly the norm for health care. Customers should be free to choose which treatment to have where and when. This presupposes that customers are well informed about available choices, are in a position mentally and emotionally to make these choices, and have the cash resources to pay for them, and also that the treatments chosen are available where and when they are wanted or needed. There are two big difficulties with this in the UK: the National Health Service (NHS) does not function as a market at present; and not all people (in fact, only a very few) have the financial resources to buy health care. An ever-widening gap of inequality is therefore appearing. There are many stories about people who have been refused treatment or given inappropriate treatments for questionable reasons:

- Women are forced to undergo Caesarean section against their will (Dimond 2001b).
- A Gallup poll in April 1999 revealed that one in 20 people aged 65 years had been refused treatment, while one in 10 has been treated differently since the age of 50 (Payne 2000a).
- A cancer patient in her 60s, despite still being in a generally good state of health, discovered that a junior doctor she had never met had put a 'do not resuscitate' order on her medical records (Payne 2000a).

- A 45-year-old mother of five young children was told that her hip operation could not be performed within the foreseeable future because the hospital's budget was overspent.

The economy–efficiency–effectiveness model for evaluating health care is akin to the analytical model of health; unless it can be measured it is of no use. Against this needs to be put the holistic model of health care that takes a wider and broader view, in which not only solutions to problems are considered but also different aspects of caring, responsibility, meaning of life and suffering, and respect for the individual.

How health care is measured is inevitably a contentious issue. The expansion of technology means that therapies and treatments are now available that were never dreamt of when the NHS was conceived. Indeed, the inventors of the NHS believed that, once everyone was healthy, it would be very cheap to run such a national service. In the last decade of the twentieth century in particular, many of the national institutions suffered a serious loss of credibility. The NHS was particularly hard hit by stories of the Bristol heart surgeons who carried on operating on children despite extremely high mortality rates; the general practitioner (GP) Dr Harold Shipman who killed dozens of elderly women and was not brought to justice for years; the pathologist at Alder Hey Children's Hospital who stored organs without parents' consent; and 'postcode prescribing' (the practice by which someone living on one side of a road would be able to receive a certain treatment, but someone living on the other side would not, because they live in different (former) health authorities). These and countless other stories and incidents reduced the level of confidence not only in medical personnel but also in their care and treatments. The market forces that apply to some degree in these incidents also gave the impression that health care is more like a lottery than an effective service. It had become possible to consult a GP and demand a treatment or medication described on a website. Viagra, the drug for male erectile dysfunction, became a battle ground of wills between the public and GPs. GPs, and nurses, became frightened, or were at least suspicious of, the 'expert patient'.

Not all treatments and possibilities are beneficial. With the great choice of therapies and treatments available it is becoming ever more difficult to make a right or even an adequate choice.

With the present fall in the number of school-leavers there will not be enough nurses to care for the growing numbers of elderly people who now need more attention to stay alive and remain independent. There are more worthwhile activities to be undertaken than there are human, material and organisational resources to support them. Resources put to one use will be taken away from another and the clash of priorities may be so strong that it could become impossible even to undertake some worthwhile activities (Weale 1988).

Against this there are also government guidelines to improve certain areas of health care, such as cancer and heart disease. These bring with them secondary needs, such as management of chronic illness and disability, particularly after stroke (Williams and Kendall 1998). Any illness has some consequences in terms of housing, job opportunities, and family stress, possibly affecting children and their schooling. Nurses cannot stand by and not consider these issues.

Should health care be rationed? John Cutliffe (1999) thinks it should, given that we do not live in an ideal world, but in one where ever increasing demand and finite resources will always clash.

Despite efforts towards equality in health care, a Social Policy Research report published by the Joseph Rowntree Foundation in 1997 shows that *where* a child is born in Britain 'is more important than ever in determining that child's life chances, particularly his or her chances of survival'. The report showed that in 'Hammersmith, Port-Glasgow and Southwark a man [aged 15–44] is more than twice as likely to die than average and in too many areas to list… adult male mortality rates are high and rising'.

To determine the priorities in health care will become an ever more acute problem. The danger is that patients eventually become objects and means to ends. Claims for excellence in one centre are likely to become and be seen to be empire-building exercises for strong personalities, and colleagues who do not get on with each other will vie over budgets and their part in them. This has probably always been the case. However, with shrinking resources, more open and more flat management, and much more public accountability, there is also more public knowledge and involvement. Economy, efficiency and effectiveness are surely useful values in health care, but only as long as they are tempered with ethics.

GLOBAL HEALTH VALUES

While the global village has opened up an exciting world to us, it has also made us aware of the misery of what is often called the 'Majority World' or the 'Two-Thirds World'. We cannot escape from the daily news of famine, floods and children suffering from diseases that could be remedied at the cost of a few pence. What we do in one part of the world affects another. Our values affect those of the poorest nations, and their plight affects not only our consciences and living standards, but needs to affect our values, and the huge contradictions in our value systems.

- Rich nations benefit from increasing technology use and people live many years longer than even 20 years ago. However, we do not care well for our older people.
- We have programmes for fertility treatment, often investing vast sums in having one baby. At the same time we ask people in poor nations to have fewer children.
- Our pharmaceutical companies develop more and more 'life-style' drugs (such as Viagra), but spend next to no money on developing drugs that would help the poorer nations to fight diseases such as malaria, tuberculosis and parasitic infestations. A related point is the case of drugs for human immunodeficiency virus/acquired immune deficiency syndrome (HIV/AIDS) in Africa, India and Central America, where drug companies had blocked nations from producing their own cheap generic drugs for many years.
- Western nations send either inappropriate drugs or drugs near to expiry dates to countries after disasters (Reich et al 1999).

Although none of this may affect any of us directly, yet it does, because these things are done by our governments in our name. It is easy to plead an inability to change the government. This may not be so any longer. While national governments seem remote and people are no longer interested in politics as such, it has become more worth while to take up a single issue. In the UK this has been the debt cancellation for poor countries issue (the Jubilee campaign), cheaper petrol in 2000, and lobbies of countryside issues, not forgetting the women of Greenham Common in the 1980s. All these campaigns have largely achieved what they set out to do.

Perhaps the single most important and growing issue world-wide is long-term care. People are living longer and become frailer, thus needing care. Some countries in Africa have become so decimated by HIV/AIDS that it is the older generation who are now caring for the younger, rather than the other way round. It is unclear who will care for *them* in their old age. In the western world families and their homes have become smaller and they are often away from other family members who may need care. Much of the burden of care world-wide falls on women, who often have less access to, or control of, the resources needed to carry out this task. Miriam Hirschfeld (2002), Special Adviser at the World Health Organization (WHO), has outlined the main ethical and human rights dimensions in this area; her questions demand that personal, professional, national and international values are all considered seriously:

- *How do societies view old, disabled, chronically ill citizens, people with malaria, TB [tuberculosis], HIV/AIDS, and why?*
- *What are the values in society with regard to taking care of disabled people?*
- *How can health and social services be prioritized and rationed, or target groups prioritized?*
- *What are the criteria for rationing and are the criteria based on need?*
- *How can resources for long-term care including home care be allocated with clearly defined priorities?*
- *Do communities have collective responsibilities?*
- *What can and should governments do to encourage and share responsibility for the development of initiatives for policy making, financing, and providing long-term care?*
- *How can roles and responsibilities be shared among clients, caregivers, families, communities, and governments?* (p. 103)

Global health care does indeed affect us all. Nurses are in strategic positions here (Miriam Hirschfeld is a nurse) and have an increasing duty to be involved in issues that are beyond their immediate surroundings of care.

VALUES OF NURSING

These far-reaching issues challenge nurses who say that they are not interested in politics or management but just want to get on with their job. *How* they get on with their job will become increasingly crucial.

Nurses are constantly affected by budgets, usually most immediately by shortage of staff. All over the NHS other shortages are evident: linen, cleaners, security personnel and dressing packs. It is possible to make do once or twice, but when the situation becomes chronic, people lose interest and their morale drops. A dispirited nurse is not going to cheer up a patient very readily. It is less and less easy to be compassionate, committed and conscientious if all around the standards are dropping. How nurses react to such situations, not just emotionally but practically, makes them ethical nurses.

Frankl (1962) believes that the most urgent task for people is to find meaning for their lives. It could be said that nursing too has to search for its meaning, again and again. The values of society change; with them the values of nursing change and each generation of nurses has to discover its own values for itself. Indeed, that nursing is so sensitive to such changes is one of its strengths.

Professional issues will always have a dominant place. Some of these will be addressed specifically in Chapter 9. Some more general concerns and values only are considered here.

It is interesting to see how professional issues have moved from the debate about whether or not nursing is a profession; whether or not nursing can be independent, and whether or not nurses can prescribe care, to the more fundamental issues about care itself. The concern is increasingly what care is, what it is meant to do or give, and who gives what care. There is also an increasing need for care to be culturally relevant.

The Health Service Ombudsman's Annual Report for 2000 lists many cases of simple neglect and, as in previous years, blames poor communication as the main problem. That Report and many other documents (e.g. the United Kingdom Central Council's *Fitness for Practice*, 1999a) carry the pious hope that there will be an improvement shortly. For this to take place it needs commitment from all concerned, and that is far from easy to implement.

The values of health care are often put in terms of value for money. Decisions have to be made in the light of this and 'depending on how compassionate and civilized we want our society to be' (Salvage 1985, p. 152). This brings us back to the wider national and international issues.

Mike Nolan and co-authors (2001) believe that 'relationship-centred care is the next logical step' (p. 757) in nursing, because person-centred care is not the most appropriate way forward. Although it has been hailed in various documents as the ideal, 'caregiving can only be fully understood within the context of a relationship' (p. 757). This is also what long-term care is about and what matters to care-givers everywhere. It is above all what an ethic of care is about.

There are no absolutely right or wrong values to hold for nurses; that would be too easy. The various values outlined in this chapter will all apply at one stage or another. All ethics means that listening and hearing is essential, be this listening to a child, a person who is lonely, or international policy makers. It is in the latter category that hearing is particularly needed. It is too easy to make policies that are useless or even harmful. Listening is the very basic skill of communication; at the basis of ethics, therefore, is communication. Thus it may be appropriate to put forward one more set of values: those of communication. This set is outlined by William Johnston (1981) as a basis for dialogue between Christians and Buddhists; that is, between people of very different cultures. However, Buddhist ideals are gaining greatly in many spheres in the West, and the leading action of Buddhism—compassion—is also a component of caring. This set therefore admirably complements the Five Cs:

- Be attentive
- Be intelligent
- Be reasonable
- Be responsible
- Be committed (Johnston 1981).

Nurses who hold any of these values care deeply and, by doing so, are not only 'just' committed to their job but are also agents of change, professionals, partners and companions.

4

Theories of ethics

ETHICS AND MORALITY

We make many ethical decisions every day, but we usually do not think if we make decisions on the basis of a particular theory or principle. We choose, prize and act upon our values, but ethics involves more reflection and argument.

The word 'ethics' comes from the Greek word *ethos*, meaning character. 'Morals' comes from the Latin word *moralis*, meaning custom, or manner. Both words mean custom (i.e. fundamental ways of conduct that are not only customary, but also right).

Being moral often implies that a person lives within a clear-cut set of personal or religious dogmas. Ethics implies transparency, public accountability, or taking a stand for or against certain public issues. Every public organisation has its code of ethics so that people can hold the organisation to account, if necessary. Clearly, ethics has become an important way of life in a postmodern society that does not acknowledge any fixed points of reference.

TWO VIEWS OF ETHICS

There are two different ways of viewing ethics: normative and descriptive.

Normative, or prescriptive, ethics is to do with norms and prescriptions: how people *should* live and behave. Codes of conduct or ethics stem from the basis of normative ethics.

The descriptive, or scientific, study of ethics has come to the fore since the advent of the social sciences. Socrates (469–399 BC) was condemned to death for his (too) rigorous pursuit of finding out what people thought and meant by words like 'justice' and 'virtue', and could therefore be called a social scientist. The studies of sociologists, anthropologists and psychologists describe what people *actually do*, uncovering areas of personal and societal behaviour. As an example, the constraints by Victorian society on sexual matters were uncovered to a large extent by sociologists who studied people's actual behaviour, not only what they said they did. Once such evidence becomes public, taboos about behaviour no longer remain taboo, and some particular behaviours pass into the area of norms. Once the majority of people think or behave in a new form, laws have to be created to accommodate this new behaviour. This in turn leads to codes that state how people ought to or should behave in certain circumstances.

The difference between descriptive and normative aspects of ethics is particularly evident in health care. The medical model tends to be concerned with the scientific and descriptive aspects of care. This model analyses illnesses, studies stress in relation to illness, divides people into classes, and compares diseases within social classes with the aim of curing disease. It is concerned with the description of ethical behaviour. This model has enabled the proliferation of high technology in medical care. The question then becomes if the ends have justified the means. There will

---

Box 4.1 Two approaches to ethics

NORMATIVE (prescriptive) (what we should do)	DESCRIPTIVE (what we actually do)
Mainly used by philosophers	Mainly used by sociologists, psychologists, anthropologists
Emphasis is on making recommendations for behaviour	Emphasis is on observation of behaviour
In health care: Pursues: • The concept of health • The significance of human suffering • Rights of patients • Dimensions of caring • Concepts, such as compassion, commitment, etc. • Meaning of death.	*In health care:* Pursues: • Psychology of illness • Physiology of stress • Social pressures in chronic disease.
Deciding whether a patient *ought* to receive a particular care	Describing *how* the treatment is best given

never be clear-cut conclusions because the means of one group are the ends of another. Thus the heart of ethics is concerned with goodness, justice and truth, and how these interrelate with each other, and with behaviour between people.

Nurses have generally concerned themselves more with the normative than the descriptive aspects of health care. They have always been involved with wider issues of health, such as the significance and meaning of suffering and death, and the role and purpose of caring and compassion. It is notable that in the field of care for dying people nurses have largely led the way. Box 4.1 sets out the two approaches to ethics.

Nurses have also been prominent in the care of people with mental illness and learning difficulties, and in other specialist care for people with long-term illnesses.

It is important to be aware of these differences, not for the sake of argument but for the complementarity of certain aspects of care, and for how each pursuit can help the other in giving the best possible holistic care.

THEORIES OF ETHICS: TWO SCHOOLS

Within normative ethics there are two broad, traditional schools that have shaped thinking down the ages in the West. Each system is complete in itself, although today it is almost impossible to declare oneself an adherent to either one of them. Only a very superficial outline is possible here.

The ethical question in both systems is: 'What is the right thing to do?' A decision therefore depends on what is meant by 'right'. Each theory gives its answer from a different point of view.

Teleology

Teleology (Greek for logic of ends), or consequentialism, is concerned about ends, goals, purposes and purposiveness. Teleological arguments are concerned with consequences and outcomes. Right is seen in terms of the good produced as the consequences of an action. Thus, an end can justify any means; sometimes it is possible to do 'wrong' to achieve 'right'. This theory was applied, for instance, when it was argued that HIV tests could be done when blood samples were taken for any other tests, to gauge the level of infection in the population as a whole.

The 'end' of a statistical certainty (and possible approach to care or cure) justified the means of taking blood for this purpose without persons' consent or knowledge.

The best-known subgroup of teleology is utilitarianism. The main exponent of this theory was John Stuart Mill (1806–1873), who followed Jeremy Bentham (1748–1832). Mill's *Utilitarianism* was first published in 1867 (Mill 1867). In it he describes the 'Greatest Happiness Principle', by arguing that one's actions are right if they promote happiness, but wrong if they produce pain. By happiness Mill meant pleasure, and by unhappiness he meant pain and the absence of pleasure. The basic tenet of utilitarianism is 'the greatest good for the greatest number'. All actions are future-orientated; morality does not depend on any duty.

The main difficulty with such a theory is how one can decide what is pleasure (i.e. the 'good' to be created), or what is pain and how to avoid it. To this end Mill established a theory of 'competent judges'. Only a person who has known 'higher' and 'lower' pleasures can judge truly. Mill forestalls any argument of what are 'higher pleasures' by saying that the pleasures of the mind are of a higher order than those of the body. To qualify this idea, he then had to introduce a difference between quality and quantity of pleasure. This is a rather unsatisfactory argument because not everyone's happiness consists of having a library of books at home. Are the people who perhaps pursue a particular sport (or even nursing) less competent judges of happiness, or less happy, than intellectuals?

Alastair Campbell (1984b) reasons that the roots of the British welfare state lie firmly in utilitarianism. He believes that the philosophy of Mill 'lay behind reforms in conditions of employment, in the prison system, public health provision, in parliamentary representation and in the status of women' (p. 45). He cites the *Report on the Sanitary Condition of the Labouring Population*, published in 1842, in which is the comment: 'It is an appalling fact that, of all born of the labouring classes in Manchester, more than fifty-seven per cent die before they attain five years of age, that is, before they can be engaged in factory labour.' The writers of the Report argued that the prevention of disease made economic sense: if people were healthy they could then work in factories. The greatest happiness in this case, therefore, is work and production, which remains the 'Protestant work ethic'.

Deontology

Deontology (Greek for 'what is due', or duty), also known as non-consequentialism, is the theory of '*rights* and duties, or what is absolutely right and wrong (as opposed to relatively good and bad). Modern ... deontology is based on unconditional respect for persons (or other forms of life) and may require doing what is right regardless of the consequences' (Boyd 1997, p. 68). In this theory, any decision depends on what the action itself 'ought' to be. This theory is sceptical about an ability to look into the future and make any decisions on the consequences of actions, so it considers the interests and rights of a person (human rights) as of primary importance, serving the cause of justice in this way.

The best-known advocate of this system of ethics was Immanuel Kant (1724–1804). 'For Kant, the moral problem is not how to be happy, but how to be worthy of happiness' (Jameton 1984, p. 147). The notion of right and wrong is fundamental, but so is duty, or obligation. The emphasis here is not so much on the action, but on the person performing the action. A good person is therefore described as someone who habitually acts rightly, and a right action is one that is done from a sense of duty. Kant was convinced that any person has the capability to reason and to act morally. What or who is good or right is then judged by another, 'higher' standard or morality. The most obvious example of such a standard is a divine command.

However, Kant also believed that, because he could not prove the existence of God, ethics and morality had to be able to stand independently and be acceptable by all people. To this end he established a set of moral rules or imperatives.

One of these imperatives is, 'Act only according to that maxim [conventional moral rule] by which you can at the same time will that it should become a universal law' (Jameton 1984, p. 147). This means, basically, that people who are about to make a moral decision need to ask themselves what is the rule authorising the act they are about to perform. At the same time, they need to consider that such a rule can become a universal rule for all human beings to follow (Johnstone 1994). This emphasises both the freedom of the individual and the duty of the one for the many. A right action is only right if it is done out of a sense of duty, and the only good thing without any qualification is a person's goodwill: the will to do what one knows to be right.

The present-day equivalent of an old sample story describing these two ethical theories is of two nurses working in a paediatric ward. One nurse is there because she has done her paediatric training, but, while doing that, she found that she does not actually enjoy working with sick children, but she has no option but to work there because she cannot find another more appealing job. Another nurse working there thoroughly enjoys her work. However, this does not help the first nurse. One nurse works there because she wants the money to go travelling, the other because she enjoys this kind of work. The second nurse has acquired a sense of civic duty. Kant, therefore, would judge this nurse as highly virtuous and the other as someone who, while doing a good job, demonstrates no moral worth in doing it. The universal rule would be to encourage everyone to work first for the good of others and then for lesser reasons.

Kant went further and evolved the supreme principle of morality, also called the practical imperative, the principle that is the highest rule (i.e. to treat every rational being, including oneself, always as an end and never as a mere means). This may need to be kept in mind when we would use others to obtain better jobs, or perhaps in research, where the results may matter more to someone than the good of the research participants.

These two theories are rarely applied to the letter now. It seems difficult to act without thinking of the consequences at all, or to act thinking only of the consequences. It is useful to be familiar with the basic ideas of such theories because, in any discussion or situation where decisions have to be made, people may start from opposing standpoints and may defend one theory or the other.

Theories of ethics are probably most useful in nursing for reflection on situations and for discussion of value formation. In a critical situation it is unlikely that any nurse will turn to a theory. Indeed, it has been shown (Cameron et al 2001, Swider et al 1985) that, however much theories and principles are taught to student nurses, they tend to make decisions 'in a manner more like virtue ethics' or indeed, as anecdotal evidence shows, on the basis of 'conscience'. However, conscience is also fostered and sharpened by knowledge, especially by discussing and talking with peers. Therefore, to learn about theories is important for focusing thought and learning the language necessary to express what conscience often finds difficult to articulate. Learning about ethical principles is the next step after becoming acquainted with theories.

PRINCIPLES OF ETHICS: 1

Theories of ethics tend to be exclusive and consistent only within their own reasoning. To make them accessible, clear principles are needed, which embody and cover the main tenets of the theories. Jacques Thiroux (1995) has established a set of five 'universal principles'. These stem from his conviction that humanitarian ethics—which he advocates as the most appropriate type of ethics—can be applied generally, but he also applies these principles to bioethics, business ethics, and environmental ethics. They are therefore more general than the principles of bioethics alone and, from this point of view, are more relevant to nursing.

Principles function like a compass; they provide the direction rather than serve as a road map. They are not rigid (as theories can be), but neither are they so flexible as to suit every whim and fancy. They will not provide the answers, but help to direct the thinking towards achieving a consensus on what ought to be done in difficult circumstances. They are not absolutes, but 'near-absolutes' (Thiroux 1995, p. 105).

Certain systems of ethics and belief function on the basis that there are absolute principles, such as the prohibition to kill; hence the stance taken by some faith communities and militant groups that abortion is always wrong. Thiroux (1995) claims that absolutes, such as 'human beings should not kill other human beings' (p. 106) need to exist as principles, but that every principle has to contain the clause 'unless there is a very strong justification'. Hence, principles can never be absolutes, but only ever near-absolutes. The absolute 'do not kill' thus becomes the basic moral principle that 'human beings should not kill other innocent human beings except in self-defence or in the defence of other innocent human beings.' The problem then becomes to define 'self-defence' and 'innocent'. For every principle, Thiroux argues, there must be exceptions and justifications because of the great variety of people and situations. Ethical dilemmas happen only when there is absolutely no alternative. In order, they are the principles of:

- The value of life
- Goodness or rightness
- Justice or fairness
- Truth telling or honesty
- Individual freedom.

These principles are interdependent, but they are described one after the other for the sake of clarity. At the end it will be possible to see how they interrelate.

The principle of the value of life

Thiroux (1995) sums up this principle in one phrase: 'Human beings should revere life and accept death' (p. 180).

Most, if not all, known systems of morality have an injunction against killing and for preserving life. Indeed this is the most basic law of ethics because, without human life, there is no ethics, or at least no study of ethics. This principle is referred to as a principle of the 'value' of life rather than the sanctity of life as it may be known in some circles or systems. 'Sanctity' refers only to human life (except in Jainism, where it covers all life), whereas 'value' of life necessarily includes all life. We can no longer claim that human life is independent of all other life on the planet. Although we can also observe some animals behaving in what seem to humans as ethical ways, this is probably more for the self-preservation of the species. It is clear that some animals also behave in 'altruistic' ways, as we know daily from dogs and horses at least. The increasing interest and concern with environmental issues also make it clear that our way of life has to be much more in harmony with all other created forms, otherwise life as we know it now may cease because of our own destructiveness. It is evident that we need to value life in its entirety.

This principle is placed first, and is held to be a near-absolute, 'because life is held both in common and uniquely by all human beings' (Thiroux 1995, p. 182). Life is the one thing all people have in common, but each person experiences it differently. The other four principles stand, therefore, in relation to this basic one.

It does not mean that life is life 'at all costs'; neither does it mean that quantity should always come before quality. People must know that they cannot be killed arbitrarily or have their life preserved without their informed consent, unless there is very strong justification. Because life is the basic 'given', which everybody has equally, it forms the fundamental premise for any discussion. Some justifications for taking human life do, however, exist. The following are some of the situations when life is not unquestionably either 'good' or to be preserved.

Abortion

If seen from the point of view of killing, this is an infringement of the principle of the value of life; if looked at from the point of view of the right of the person, one needs to ask: What is meant by killing, and what is meant by preserving life? Whose life is more important: the mother's or the child's? When does life begin, or at what stage does a conceptus have human life? What are the economic or health considerations that may be involved? Is rape or incest always a reason for an abortion? What is the right to life of malformed fetuses?

Most nurses have few opportunities in their working lives to encounter these issues directly, except perhaps in personal circumstances. However, they form part of their ethical stance or system and nurses may be approached for help with decision making. In each situation the issues differ and not all issues can be addressed by a few questions.

Abortion is discussed further in Chapter 8.

Euthanasia

Advances in medical technology and science have largely created this issue for medicine, nursing and the law. It is possible to keep people alive long beyond all previous expectations; thus the question becomes urgent concerning if steps should be taken to end such a life. Who should decide? Distinctions are made between voluntary and involuntary euthanasia, and letting someone die. Unlike abortion, this is an issue with which nurses grapple every day, and that perhaps causes the most ethical and professional problems.

Euthanasia is discussed in more detail in Chapter 8.

Killing in self-defence

This issue qualifies the principle of the value of life in stating that one should never kill other human beings except when defending innocent people, including oneself. The essence of this argument is that, by threatening to kill or by killing others, perpetrators, in a sense, forfeit their right to have their own lives considered as valuable.

War

War and guerrilla operations are perhaps the most powerful threats to life in general. After the events of 11 September 2001 in America, attacks against any force or regime must be analysed carefully because they may be making far more than self-interested and/or national statements. Many nurses are not only caught up in such situations but they care for the injured of both sides. Nurses working for humanitarian organisations such as Médecins Sans Frontières, which send personnel to places of conflict, often encounter situations of astonishing horror and bravery.

Capital punishment

It can be argued that capital punishment amounts to murder by society of one of its members. It can also be a form of societal revenge but, in a civilised society, revenge should not be a valid motive for taking human life. Increasing numbers of countries have abolished capital punishment for all crimes, especially for minors, with the notable exception in the west of the USA.

Suicide

Suicide is both killing and taking human life, but it is not generally considered either civilly or criminally unlawful. Thiroux (1995) states that 'most people ... would probably urge the use of all possible means to prevent people from killing themselves' (p. 207). People who support the morality of suicide would do so from a position of allowing greater freedom for individual decision making. Those who argue that suicide is always immoral 'might advocate the use of physical and legal restraints for people who are known to be suicidal' (p. 207). These scenarios may need to be discussed particularly in the mental health field, but they are issues for every nurse, whether working in hospital or the community, increasingly so for school nurses.

To whom is life a good? Moral dilemmas are caused because issues of good and right, justice, truth and personal freedom conflict, and are valued differently. This is particularly evident when the theory of quality-adjusted life-years (QALYs) (Harris 1987) is considered. Andrew Edgar and colleagues (1998) try to answer what a QALY is by saying that:

The outcomes of healthcare come in many different forms and guises. Pain relief, anxiety reduction, mobility improvement and life extension are all examples of successful outcomes of healthcare ... The basic thinking behind the QALY is that health has two main dimensions: length and quality. Effective healthcare must either extend life or improve its quality or preferably both, so in theory all effective healthcare will produce Quality Adjusted Life Years' (p. xi).

A QALY is an instrument for rationing health care that does not seem to be widely known among nurses, but all nurses are aware of some practice of rationing, even if they do not know its source or theory. Nurses and carers are faced with issues of life and death every day. It is therefore important to know both one's own value bases and also those of the person cared for. We should revere life, but also accept that it is not limitless. Who makes what decisions for people's lives and death, and on what basis, is an increasingly urgent debate, and one in which nurses must also become more involved.

The principle of goodness or rightness

This principle must logically be prior to the remaining principles because the question of good and right is basic in ethics.

Many policies, guidelines and working theories are built on the assumption that everyone has, or should have, the same understanding of values or what to consider as good. Some of the well-known goods often cited are 'life, consciousness, pleasure, happiness, truth, knowledge, beauty, love, friendship, self-expression, self-realization, freedom, honour, peace and so on' (Thiroux 1995, p. 183). These elements depend on each other, particularly on the interpretation we put on them in certain circumstances. As society changes, so its values change, and with it what it values as good or worthy of pursuit.

For an ill person, health is likely to be a good, but this concept may represent different aspects for a person who has a broken nose compared with someone who has to learn to live with multiple sclerosis. Individuals have the freedom to place more emphasis on one good or another, so it does not mean that others' goods are devalued.

'Good' should not only be in the abstract but it should be seen in relation to (other) human beings. As an example, a person who is suicidal may no longer value his or her life as a 'good', but that person's mother may have a very different concept of the value of her child's life. An artist may place a very high value of beauty on a particular painting, seeing 'beauty' as something inherent in the painting without having to justify it. Art critics may not interpret the painting in the same way.

It is not possible to talk of an ethic of care if one cannot see 'good' in relation to people, that is, in the way care is given. Thiroux (1995) argues that a sadist may gain pleasure (his 'good') by mistreating another human being. William Frankena (1973, p. 91), who treated the subject of good and right extensively, argues that there should also be 'some kind or degree of excellence' present with good actions. The person who performs a good action, who 'does a good job', should also be a 'good' person so that the action is indeed good, or that there is excellence present. Harmony and creativity are also related to good. Something that is creative or can help people to become creative also helps to bring about integration, so surely it must also be seen to be right action.

This principle demands that:

• we promote goodness over badness
• we cause no harm or badness
• we prevent badness or harm.

When actively doing good may not be possible, then doing as little harm as possible should be the aim.

In much of medicine and nursing, 'harm' has to be done in order to make people better. An operation is 'harmful', but it prevents more serious harm from the disease. Even giving an injection is potentially harmful. In order to prevent harm from treatments and care, it is therefore important that policies and guidelines concerning procedures are followed. This means also that good teaching should take place concerning equipment use, moving and handling patients, and taking safety precautions. Much of this seems no more than common sense, but, as noted above, rationalisation and scarce resources can lead to much cutting of corners, and all health-care personnel have duties to ensure that, when the best is not possible, at least no harm is caused. What they do about any danger signs, and how successful they are in raising standards, is not only a matter of professional duty, but also of ethical 'excellence'. In this way, good people perform right actions.

The principle of justice or fairness

'It is not enough that people should try to be good and do what is right; there must also be some attempt made to distribute the benefits from being good and doing right' (Thiroux 1995, p. 184). The ethical questions are: who should receive the benefits from good human actions and how should they be distributed?

It is not the moral assumptions underlying medical ethics that are disputed, but the application of these assumptions to specific cases is a different matter. When certain treatments are available to some people, but not to others, the notion of justice becomes urgent. Nurses have written very little about distributive justice in health care. However, in many countries, nurses are actively 'doing' justice in accident and emergency departments. When resources are limited, is a treatment given to people on the basis of:

- Who deserves it?
- Who needs it?
- Who is able in the long run to make most use of it?
- Who has been on the waiting list longest?

The question of need is almost ruled out because presumably everyone needs that particular treatment if they have this particular complaint.

- Who decides who is to live, and how much value persons should place on their life?

The classic example tends to be organ transplants. There are far more people with stated needs for a transplant than there are organs available. How can one part of the population be persuaded that what they potentially can give is to be used for another part of the population? How do we ensure that health is not simply a personal matter, but is a social concern where those who have more share with those who have less? In all European countries the willingness to donate organs has declined. Perhaps this is not surprising after the various cases of misappropriation of organs that have become public. However, a kidney transplant is much cheaper in the long run than dialysis. Should an economic (or monetary) criterion be added to the information that potential organ donors are given; or should some value statement be made on donor cards carried by people to the effect that we are responsible to and for each other as a society? The distribution of scarce resources will remain an issue of justice, but:

- Do we judge according to the individual right of the person, or how much can be saved by one procedure over another?
- Does the end (saving money for other procedures) justify the means (not giving one particular treatment)?

The most ethical, just and fair way to determine who benefits from limited resources may be a fairly conducted lottery. However, health should not depend on a lottery, but on some good reason. The increasing emphasis on the market and the ideals of being consumers means that we have become used to having what we want, and we want it now. This is the case not only for consumer goods, but also for health care. As a society we have become impatient with inefficiency and with waiting. We have also learned that if we cannot get something by asking for it nicely, we can get it by going to the press and making a fuss.

We also argue that discrimination on the grounds of merit, ability, age, race, status, or anything else, is not acceptable. If we suspect any discrimination, we make it known, perhaps citing a particular code or mission statement. Any issue of justice or equality is difficult to apply. We need to 'recognize the common equality of human beings as human beings and yet allow for individual differences in attempting to distribute goodness and badness fairly' (Thiroux 1995, p. 185). It may mean that, when confronted with the impossibility of upholding this principle, we strive at least to do no harm.

The principle of truth telling or honesty

Communication is the vehicle for ethics. In order for this to be sustained, it has to be based on truthfulness or honesty. Truth telling is therefore fundamental to being ethical and moral. If morality depends on agreements between human beings, then there must be some assurance that they are entered into and maintained honestly and truthfully (Thiroux 1995, p. 186).

Yet, this principle is probably the most difficult one to maintain or to live. Human relationships of any kind are delicate and, to protect their own vulnerability in this area, people have built up defences against exposing themselves to others. Being economical with the truth is only one way of putting this. A quick glance at any thesaurus will reveal that in our language there are fewer synonyms for truth than for untruth or deception.

Every nurse knows how important this principle is. Every treatment or care depends on truth revealed and a response made. Symptoms need to be accurately described or elicited and treated accordingly. However, communication goes further than facts. What is said or not said between people can drastically affect a person's mind and lead to further health or illness. The difficulty is that 'the truth' is not simply a fact, but also a process, growing and developing, leading to insight and coming from experience.

Henry David Thoreau (1849) wrote that: 'it takes two to speak the truth,—one to speak, and another to hear' (p. 697). It is this aspect of hearing that is crucial for the telling of truth. How clients or patients perceive their truth may be more important than that we give them our truth.

Communication that is intended to be truly helpful may require preparation, and telling the truth may not just be a matter of making a factual statement. Particularly when 'bad news' has to be given to someone (by which we usually mean a diagnosis of cancer or a foreshortened life), *how* this news is given is as important as that it *is* given, and by *whom*.

This can be illustrated by the story of Harry:

Harry was 11 when he was admitted with a painful and swollen left leg, diagnosed as sarcoma. Harry lived with his younger sister and recently divorced mother. On the ward he was quiet but watched every game of football and rugby on the television. His mother had been adamant that Harry should not be told anything of his prognosis and the consultant had agreed to this. Harry had suffered quite enough already, she said. Clare, a student nurse, became very friendly with Harry and he asked her more and more questions about his leg, which she found increasingly difficult to answer because of the proviso not to tell him anything. She asked that this 'don't tell policy' should be reversed, but the consultant felt he could not let Harry's mother down. Clare decided she could not maintain her integrity under these circumstances and asked to be transferred to another ward. Harry became quiet and withdrawn again, and died 3 weeks later.

This story is complicated because Harry is a minor and his mother's wishes have to be respected. It is accepted today that children should be involved in their care as much as possible, giving consent where indicated. As a student nurse, Clare may not have had the confidence to challenge the mother's request; however, both she and the mother may have needed support from a colleague who was competent in dealing with issues of family relationships.

It is clearly very necessary to be aware of cultural needs and expectations and respect these. In some cultures, telling someone they have cancer is regarded as being extremely insensitive. Chinese people may never again trust a doctor who tells them that they have cancer; just the opposite may be the case in the UK.

The following is an account of events with a tragic outcome. One wonders if truth had been spoken but never heard: M L looked after her 25-year-old son (who had severe Down's syndrome) alone after her husband was killed in a road accident. When she was operated on after several months of feeling tired and nauseated, she was told that a great deal of liquid had been removed from her abdomen. She was told that she needed to rest her intestine, and that she would have some chemotherapy 'as a precaution'. She was not particularly curious about her illness, and went home, anxious to look after her son, not suspecting that she had advanced carcinoma of the ovary. When she continued to vomit, she was told she had overstretched her liver; when she became breathless, that she had bronchitis. She died, unable to make any provision for her son.

Martin Benjamin and Joy Curtis (1986) think that 'a person of integrity … is one whose responses to various matters are not capricious or arbitrary, but principled. One of the qualities most of us admire in others and try to cultivate in ourselves is personal integrity' (p. 17).

The same authors point out that any act of deception or untruth has a corrosive effect on the relationships that are necessary to maintain social bonds. This is particularly true in nursing and medicine. It is therefore all the more surprising that both nursing and medical codes of professional conduct have traditionally been mute on the subject of truthfulness. However, the Nursing and Midwifery Council Code (2002) states in clause 3.1 that registered nurses and midwives should give information that is 'accurate, truthful and presented in such as way as to make it easily understood'. This is a welcome addition to this important text for UK nursing.

Deception, wrote Benjamin and Curtis (1986) 'is a form of manipulation, and manipulation, like coercion and rational persuasion, is a way of inducing others to do what one wants them to do' (p. 62). It corrodes trust by making light of truth, and that in turn is destructive to helping and caring relationships.

Issues of conflicting claims can be difficult to handle. When nurses do not know who has the greatest claim on their time, skill or attention, they may have to resort to manipulative or underhand practices. The patient usually has the greatest claim, but various members of the family (particularly in the case of child patients) or doctors make equally strong claims on nurses' professional and emotional capacities. Nurses' loyalty is to their patients because they care for them, but they also respect the family, a unit that may have functioned for years in a particular way and which they have no right to destroy.

In a case conference discussed by Roger Higgs (1985) of a situation similar to that of Harry, most of the commentators suggested that the adults (parents and doctors) should be given an opportunity to voice their fears, angers and worries. The point was made strongly that: 'When we think we can tell them what's wrong, then we're missing the point. We have to find out what they are worried about … One has to understand … by listening to [them] and not spend hours talking at [them]' (p. 157). An ethic of caring essentially listens and, in listening, 'hears' the people and their problems; by doing that, 'problems' may already be reduced and trust restored.

When various occupational groups are willing to trust each other, a great deal of energy is freed up for more essential work, time is saved, duplication is reduced, and patient care is improved. Daniel Chambliss (1996) also observed that, in hospital, many, if not all, 'ethical problems are an expression of interest group conflict' (p. 11). 'Partnering' is the approach described by David Nicholson (2000), that has been used in the public and private sectors with good effect, removing professional boundaries and stereotypes. There is plenty of scope to address and face these issues with honesty and truth in the whole of health care.

The principle of individual freedom

Like life, freedom is 'built into' the human structure. Freedom, however, is a matter of morality; we need to use freedom to preserve life, do right and be good, act justly and tell the truth. If we had no freedom to do this, or to reject it, there would be no morality. Therefore, neither this principle nor the other four can stand alone.

Each person is unique, and individually will (and should) express the first four principles in a unique way. We may not be social or economic equals, but we are all moral equals, however much some people's lifestyles differ. However, moral decisions often differ because of individual variations in upbringing and life experiences.

Individual freedom is not simply something that is given; we need to use that freedom in order to be fully functioning individuals. Both deontology and teleology put less emphasis on freedom than on the necessity to choose rightly. Freedom is not a licence to do as we please; it is freedom to act morally. The freedom exists to pick up something displayed in a shop, but moral freedom prevents us from stealing it.

We have freedom in the way we behave to each other and to society: how we educate our children, who we choose as friends, how we use the money we earn, what books and magazines we read. Moral and ethical behaviour is seen in the consequences of any of these acts. The dilemma arises, as already mentioned, because many of our personal acts affect society. Can we—or to what extent can or should we—believe that we have the right to choose on any matter and let the state pick up the consequences? An ethic of care starts from a different angle. It does not prescribe or moralise; it simply points out that to care is to be human, and that the human mode of being is to care. We care for each other personally and we have a responsibility socially. The freedom of the individual is not curtailed by this. Rather, it is enhanced because the choice to care means that this and the other principles mentioned here are seen as being governed by receptivity, relatedness and responsiveness.

If we had no freedom, we could not be moral. It is therefore possible to see that, with this last principle, how all the others interact and are necessary to each other. If one of the principles falls, they all fall like dominoes. If we tell a lie, we do not act as good persons; other people in turn cannot act rightly; we devalue the other person and overvalue ourselves, thus reducing justice; our freedom to be moral is restricted because, once embarked on the course of a lie, we have to continue on it, thus perpetuating the deception. This principle of individual freedom is therefore essential in any system of principles. In health care it is particularly necessary because there we are confronted with people at vulnerable points in their lives, often needing to make delicate decisions. They need to be assisted and encouraged when possible, not coerced, in order to satisfy their own needs. That this is far from easy is evident by how much we are influenced by the media and advertising. We are told every day that we 'need' this or that for life, that our own thoughts may be crowded out, and making our own decisions can become problematic. This is all the more reason why we need to be sensitive to people's needs to be themselves in the 'moments of truth' that illnesses or accidents often become.

PRINCIPLES OF ETHICS: 2

The best-known approach to ethics within medicine is that propagated by Tom Beauchamp and James Childress in their book *Principles of Biomedical Ethics* (2001). They took their approach from the Belmont Report (President's Commission 1981), which was the outcome of the National Commission for the Protection of Human Subjects of Biomedical and Behavioral Research, which was established in 1973 in the USA to draw up regulations that should protect the rights and interests of participants in research. The Belmont Report considered that respect for persons, beneficence and justice should be the ethical principles governing research. Beauchamp and Childress added the principle of non-maleficence (doing no harm), thus making these the four principles that have come to be associated with medical ethics:

- Respect for autonomy
- Non-maleficence
- Beneficence
- Justice.

The differences between this set of principles and the foregoing ones are perhaps mostly in appearance, but this set lacks the specific mention of truth telling or honesty. However, denoting a specific principle as doing no harm is also specific here. Theories of ethics would claim that actually 'doing good' takes priority over simply avoiding harm. William Frankena (1973) makes the distinction between having a duty to oneself or only to others. If one has a duty to oneself, then beneficence comes first; if to others, then non-maleficence has precedence.

Raanan Gillon (1986), as perhaps the best-known defender of the four principles in the UK, wrote that:

While it seems entirely plausible to claim that we owe non-maleficence, but not beneficence, to everybody, it does not follow from this that avoidance of doing harm (non-maleficence) takes priority over beneficence. All that follows is that the scope of non-maleficence is general, encompassing all other people, whereas the scope of beneficence is more specific, applying only to some people (p. 81).

In many instances in nursing and medicine, non-maleficence is certainly more applicable than beneficence. Life is risky, often leading to illness and accidents; and treatments, operations and medications all cause 'harm' in the interest of health. One can therefore argue that regaining one's health is also risky, but the risks should not be worse than the benefits gained. Doing no harm is therefore an important principle because it keeps before practitioners' minds the obligation to practice their skill with every respect.

The difference between autonomy and individual freedom is subtle. Gillon (1986) writes of autonomy of thought, autonomy of will (or perhaps intention), and autonomy of action. This seems to emphasise a rather intellectual approach to freedom. Thiroux (1995) appears to have a somewhat more holistic stance when he wrote that, although human beings 'have common characteristics (bodies, minds, feelings, and so forth), each person is, nevertheless, unique' (p. 188). People's needs, desires and concerns vary greatly; to acknowledge them and accommodate them, there needs to be freedom (autonomy), but a freedom bounded by other principles.

The principle of respect for autonomy (or the person) is perhaps more specific than the principle of the value of life. Respect for the person is rooted in the desire to avoid suffering, but doing precisely this can interfere with another's freedom. Respect for others is an essential ethical principle and task, but it is not to be used exclusively, that is, respecting only the person of the patient to the exclusion of the individual's group of supporters or carers.

This set of principles has been associated in particular with bioethics, which is an interdisciplinary field. It includes medicine, nursing, the biomedical sciences, law, economics and public policy, as well as the work of philosophers and religious thinkers, whose domain ethics had almost exclusively been until bioethics arrived (Kuhse and Singer 1998).

Bioethics has held the field of health care more or less unchallenged for many years. It has spread all over the world, and nurses in many countries have been nurtured on the famous four principles, perhaps rather unquestioningly. As mentioned in chapter 1, this is no longer the case.

Other approaches to ethics in health care

In recent years many other approaches to ethics generally, and within nursing in particular, have been written about and used, both theoretically and practically. Some of them are addressed in detail in the companion volume to this book *Approaches to Ethics: Nursing Beyond Boundaries* (Tschudin, 2003). They are therefore mentioned here only for interest.

Care ethics is used and described in this current volume.

Virtue ethics has greatly influenced nursing in recent years and therefore needs a mention here.

It has been argued that virtue ethics has gained in importance because of the dissatisfaction with some aspects of mainstream theories of ethics (Oakley 1998). Like an ethic of care, virtue ethics does not start with certain principles into which ethical problems need to fit; the main criterion is what sort of a person one ought to be and what sort of life one ought to live.

Instead of considering 'right', 'wrong', 'obligations' or what is 'permissible', virtue ethics approaches challenge in terms of being 'courageous', 'honest', 'just' or 'callous', according to Justin Oakley (1998, p. 86). Alasdair MacIntyre (1985) considers several virtues within cultures and history in his famous book, *After Virtue*, writing about them in detail. Oakley lists six key claims that are essential to virtue ethics:

- *An action is right if and only if it is what an agent with a virtuous character would do in the circumstances.* Virtue ethics starts with the character. Perhaps the main question in this theory is why someone would want to be a good person and do good actions.
- *Goodness is prior to rightness.* This is also necessary in other theories of ethics, but here it is fundamental; the person matters before the action.
- *The virtues are irreducibly plural intrinsic goods.* The virtues cannot

be reduced to just one value, but various virtues are necessary for good actions, such as honesty, courage, loyalty. In other words, a fully functioning human being can be so at many levels.

- *The virtues are objectively good.* The virtues are good independently of any connections of any particular desire or ethical situation.
- *Some intrinsic goods are agent relative.* Some theories of ethics claim that 'good' is independent of a person (agent), but virtue ethics considers that every action depends on the person.
- *Acting rightly does not require that we maximise the good.* Some theories argue that only the best is good enough in any ethics. Virtue ethics, however, looks for 'excellence'. Oakley (1998) states that instead of looking only for the best friendships, we should instead look for 'excellent' friendships.

Virtues are the crux here, so Oakley makes the important point, relevant to the subject of this book, that 'doctors [and nurses] ought to tell the truth, not so much because of the importance of informed consent and respect for patient autonomy, but rather because that is what is involved in their having the virtue of truthfulness' (p. 93). In this theory, as also in an ethic of care, integrity is a main element. When considering the often conflicting claims of personal, professional and social demands, it is vital that self-awareness is practised, because integrity is what keeps a person sane when pulled in many directions.

Narrative ethics

The use of stories to create ethical reasoning is described by Anne Bishop and John Scudder (1996) and by Robin Lindsay and Helen Graham (2000).

Casuistry (case approach)

A particular case is taken as a basis for making decisions in similar cases. John Arras (1998) has written on this topic.

Feminine and feminist approaches

These approaches consider the aspects that concern women in particular. Nel Noddings (1984), and Helen Holmes and Laura Purdy (1992) have contributed to the study of this approach.

Culturally sensitive ethics

Taking issues that are relevant to a specific culture or people is becoming increasingly popular. Sandy Haegert (2000) has written movingly on this topic.

Human rights approaches

Human rights are used as a study tool for the wider learning and teaching of ethics. (*Nursing Ethics* 2001, the whole issue).

Service ethics

In this approach primacy is given to contractual relationships in service. There is a recognition of reciprocal rights and duties. This approach stresses private accountability and confidentiality, with special emphasis on respect for persons and justice (Thompson et al 2000).

Public office ethics

Here, primacy is given to service of the common good in recognition of reciprocal rights and duties, and acceptance of public accountability, with special emphasis on justice and equity through a community participation and welfare focus (Thompson et al 2000).

NIEBUHR'S RESPONSE ETHICS

This theory is not so much an alternative as another way of expressing basic tenets. H Richard Niebuhr's theory of responsibility is a means of putting the concept of relationship into an ethical framework.

Niebuhr (1963) points out that deontology asks, 'What is the law?' ('What ought I to do?') Thus we recognise the citizen. Teleology asks, 'What is the goal?' In this we recognise the maker. Response ethics asks, 'What is happening?', and so we recognise the answerer: the person who responds. This points to the basic premise that people are responsive, creative persons. All our actions are a response to actions upon us and our interpretations of these actions. Through listening we hear (we interpret) and then we respond. We respond 'to challenge rather than from the pursuit of an ideal or from adherence to some ultimate law' (Niebuhr 1963 p. 59).

This theory has many elements of the aspects outlined in Chapters 1 and 2. Niebuhr starts with the premise that to 'know thyself' is basic to all human functioning; by every activity we decide, choose and commit ourselves. This rests on the further premise that what we all have in common is our humanity. This stresses co-humanity and community: in order to stay within humanity we have to act humanly. How we interpret that humanity colours our actions. We are creative and responsive persons, so this means that we need freedom in order to be creative, and, with fidelity to that creativity, we answer responsibly. Responding and responsibility therefore complement each other.

Niebuhr outlines the pattern that takes place when we respond to an *ethical challenge*, which can be anything that makes us stop and think what *response* to give. The challenge can be having to undergo an abortion, or making or receiving an awkward telephone call. The challenge can be a major life event or a small interaction; both demand a response. Often the first response is a physical one: the heart beats faster; the mouth becomes dry; the knees become weak. This response is caused by memories from previous similar situations. The memories have stayed with us, either as fearful events, or because of our inability to deal with the situation effectively. Our response to the challenge is an *interpreted* action upon us. The challenge needs to be interpreted for the present. Hence, Niebuhr argues, every response is made in response to something or someone, as we interpret what we have heard or experienced. So that we can make the fitting response, and on the basis of 'What is going on?' we then become *accountable* to the future. We interpret the past for the future through accountability. We respond; we give the fitting answer. When the response is fitting, there is *social solidarity*. The outcome is good, or at least satisfactory, for everyone. This is what takes place naturally when there is conscious decision making based on the two main questions that Niebuhr considers are essential:

- What is happening?
- What is the fitting answer?

The pattern therefore is:

- The ethical challenge:
  —Response
    —Interpretation
      —Accountability
        —Social solidarity.

At every level, the question, 'What is happening?' is crucial. It is possible to say that this is perhaps the simplest question ever to ask, but also the one least often asked. In a difficult situation we are more inclined to ask, 'What must I do?' or 'What should I say?' Rather than jump to conclusions and make assumptions about people and situations, a far more ethical line to take is to ask the person or persons concerned, ourselves, the situation itself, and everyone else. However, as has been pointed out so often already, asking is not enough. The ethical act is the listening, the hearing, and acting on what has been heard. The question, 'What is happening?' needs to be asked, but above all it has to be answered and heard. This is where Niebuhr's responsibility comes in.

The second question, 'What is the fitting answer?' will be answered when the first question has been thoroughly asked and answered. It is significant that, in this ethic, it is the 'fitting' answer that is looked for, rather than the 'right', 'correct' or 'dutiful' answer. The answer given is the one that is fitting for the persons and the situation concerned. It is not an arbitrary answer, but one based on all the elements that make up an ethical challenge.

This theory seems particularly apt for nursing because it is not simply abstract. In nursing there is a continuum of relationships and, if care is to be given at all, it depends on relationships. How these relationships function shows how we respond, how we interpret actions upon us and respond further. Both deontology and teleology tend to come from the isolated standpoint of the individual who is concerned only with the self: 'What ought I to do?' and 'What is my aim?' Response ethics stresses the relational aspect, which asks 'What is happening and with whom?' This question looks for more details and further enquiry so as to see a greater whole and more aspects of the same problem in order to respond more responsibly. It helps to eliminate the assumptions we make and take for granted about people and situations, and enables us to act ethically.

The elements of this approach to ethics will be used in later chapters to enhance the ethic of care.

There are plenty of other approaches to ethics being used, and new ones will inevitably emerge in time, and be tried and tested.

5

Codes and declarations

CODES

Normative, or prescriptive, ethics (see Ch. 4) is concerned with interpreting philosophical statements and theories. It is not enough to put a set of ideals before people; guidelines of ideals and theories need to be transferable into action. Codes are not laws; in a sense they come before the law. The Ten Commandments, the Hippocratic Oath, the Highway Code and the Nursing and Midwifery Council (NMC) *Code of Professional Conduct* (2002) are all examples of such codes. They do not state or declare the obvious; they point to what should be.

Codes of practice are necessary in institutions and organisations where public accountability demands transparency. A code of practice is the instrument most accessible to the staff and the public.

Stephen Pattison (2001) has argued that codes within health and social care are not so helpful as they could be because most of them do not declare the values on which the statements are based. The United Kingdom Central Council (UKCC) *Code of Professional Conduct* (1992a) needed the two supplementary UKCC documents, *The Scope of Professional Practice* (1992b) and *Guidelines for Professional Practice* (1996), to fill in the details in the gaps left in the Code. The NMC *Code of Professional Conduct* (2002) combines the three documents and refers to the headings of the clauses as values, which are then elaborated in the subclauses. These values are recognised as essential by all the eight main health profession regulators in the UK (i.e. pharmacists; veterinary surgeons; medical practitioners; dentists; opticians; osteopaths; chiropractors; and nurses, midwives and health visitors (a ninth, professions supplementary to medicine, is usually added to this list)).

The ideal code will perhaps never exist; codes have, after all, to satisfy a vast number of people and interests. This short chapter looks at some of the issues involved.

Main codes in nursing

The main codes for nurses practising in the UK are:

- The International Council of Nurses (ICN) *Code of Ethics for Nurses* (2000)
- The NMC *Code of Professional Conduct* (2002).

THE ICN CODE OF ETHICS FOR NURSES

The ICN Code is remarkable in its brevity. It sets out very simply what the underlying values of nursing are in detailing the four fundamental responsibilities: to promote health, to prevent illness, to restore health, and to alleviate suffering. It is also remarkable that these values have changed only little in the 50 years since the Code was first written and through the subsequent editions. Given the incredible variation of the nursing role over time, in different countries and continents, this is a really useful document. By stressing the responsibilities of nurses, the Code is formative (i.e. it aims to form the character of nurses and nursing) and it does this with a lightness of touch that is admirable.

The text of the ICN Code of Ethics for Nurses (2000) is reprinted below with the permission of the International Council of Nurses.

THE INTERNATIONAL COUNCIL OF NURSES *CODE OF ETHICS FOR NURSES*

An international code of ethics was first adopted by the International Council of Nurses (ICN) in 1953. It has been revised and reaffirmed at various times since; most recently with this review and revision completed in 2000.

Preamble

Nurses have four fundamental responsibilities: to promote health, to prevent illness, to restore health and to alleviate suffering. The need for nursing is universal.

Inherent in nursing is respect for human rights, including the right to life, to dignity and to be treated with respect. Nursing care is unrestricted by considerations of age, colour, creed, culture, disability or illness, gender, nationality, politics, race or social status.

Nurses render health services to the individual, the family and the community and coordinate their services with those of related groups.

The Code

The *ICN Code of Ethics for Nurses* has four principle elements that outline the standards of ethical conduct.

1. Nurses and people

The nurse's primary professional responsibility is to people requiring nursing care.

In providing care, the nurse promotes an environment in which the human rights, values, customs and spiritual beliefs of the individual, family and community are respected.

The nurse ensures that the individual receives sufficient information on which to base consent for care and related treatment.

The nurse holds in confidence personal information and uses judgement in sharing this information.

The nurse shares with society the responsibility for initiating and supporting action to meet the health and social needs of the public, in particular those of vulnerable populations.

The nurse also shares responsibility to sustain and protect the natural environment from depletion, pollution, degradation and destruction.

2. Nurses and practice

The nurse carries personal responsibility and accountability for nursing practice and for maintaining competence by continual learning.

The nurse maintains a standard of personal health such that the ability to provide care is not compromised.

The nurse uses judgement in relation to individual competence when accepting and delegating responsibility.

The nurse at all times maintains standards of personal conduct which reflect well on the profession and enhance public confidence.

The nurse, in providing care, ensures that the use of technology and scientific advances are compatible with the safety, dignity and rights of people.

3. Nurses and the profession

The nurse assumes the major role in determining and implementing acceptable standards of clinical nursing practice, management, research and education.

The nurse is active in developing a core of research-based professional knowledge.

The nurse, acting through the professional organisation, participates in creating and maintaining equitable social and economic working conditions in nursing.

4. Nurses and co-workers

The nurse sustains a cooperative relationship with co-workers in nursing and other fields.

The nurse takes appropriate action to safeguard individuals when their care is endangered by a co-worker or any other person.

Suggestions for use of the ICN *Code of Ethics for Nurses*

The ICN *Code of Ethics for Nurses* is a guide for action based on social needs and values. It will have meaning only as a living document if applied to the realities of nursing and health care in a changing society.

To achieve its purpose the *Code* must be understood, internalized and used by nurses in all aspects of their work. It must be available to students and nurses throughout their study and work lives.

Applying the elements of the ICN *Code of Ethics for Nurses*

The four elements of the *Code of Ethics for Nurses*: nurses and people, nurses and practice, nurses and co-workers and nurses and the profession, give a framework for the standards of conduct. The following chart will assist nurses to translate the standards into action. Nurses and nursing students can therefore:

- Study the standards under each element of the *Code*.
- Reflect on what each standard means to you. Think about how you can apply ethics in your nursing domain; practice, education, research or management.
- Discuss the *Code* with coworkers and others.
- Use a specific example from experience to identify ethical dilemmas and standards of conduct as outlined in the *Code*. Identify how you would resolve the dilemma.
- Work in groups to clarify ethical decision making and reach a consensus on standards of ethical conduct.
- Collaborate with your national nurses' association, coworkers and others in the continuous application of ethical standards in nursing practice, education, management and research.

Table 1 Element of the Code #1: Nurses and People

Practitioners and Managers
- Provide care that respects human rights and is sensitive to the values, customs and beliefs of people.
- Provide continuing education in ethical issues.
- Provide sufficient information to permit informed consent and the right to choose or refuse treatment.
- Use recording and information management systems that ensure confidentiality.
- Develop and monitor environmental safety in the workplace.

Educators and Researchers
- In curriculum include references to human rights, equity, justice and solidarity as the basis for access to care.
- Provide teaching and learning opportunities for ethical issues and decision making.
- Provide teaching and learning opportunities related to informed consent.
- Introduce into curriculum concepts of privacy and confidentiality.
- Sensitise students to the importance of social action in current concerns.

National Nurses' Associations
- Develop Position Statements and guidelines that support human rights and ethical standards.
- Lobby for involvement of nurses in ethics review committees.
- Provide guidelines, position statements and continuing education related to informed consent.
- Incorporate issues of confidentiality and privacy into a national code of ethics for nurses.
- Advocate for a safe and healthy environment.

Table 2 Element of the Code #2: Nurses and Practice

Practitioners and Managers
- Establish standards of care and a work setting that promotes quality care.
- Establish systems for professional appraisal, continuing education and systematic renewal of licensure to practice.
- Monitor and promote the personal health of nursing staff in relation to their competence for practice.

Educators and Researchers
- Provide teaching and learning opportunities that foster life-long learning and competence for practice.
- Conduct and disseminate research that shows links between continual learning and competence to practice.
- Promote the importance of personal health and illustrate its relation to other values.

National Nurses' Associations
- Provide access to continuing education through journals, conferences, distance education etc.
- Lobby to ensure continuing education opportunities and quality care standards.
- Promote healthy lifestyles for nursing professionals. Lobby for healthy work places and services for nurses.confidentiality.

Table 3 Element of the Code #3: Nurses and the Profession

Practitioners and Managers
- Set standards for nursing practice, research, education and management.
- Foster work place support of the conduct, dissemination and utilization of research related to nursing and health.
- Promote participation in national nurses' associations so as to create favourable socio-economic conditions for nurses.

Educators and Researchers
- Provide teaching/learning opportunities in setting standards for nursing practice, research, education and management.
- Conduct, disseminate and utilize research to advance the nursing profession.
- Sensitize learners to the importance of professional nursing associations.

National Nurses' Associations
- Collaborate with others to set standards for nursing education, practice, research and management.
- Develop position statements, guidelines and standards related to nursing research.
- Lobby for fair social and economic working conditions in nursing. Develop position statements and guidelines in workplace issues and other resources to support the socio-economic welfare of nurses.

Table 4 Element of the Code #4: Nurses and Co-Workers

Practitioners and Managers
- Create awareness of specific and overlapping functions and the potential for interdisciplinary tensions.
- Develop workplace systems that support common professional ethical values and behaviour.
- Develop mechanisms to safeguard the individual, family or community when their care is endangered by health care personnel.

Educators and Researchers
- Develop understanding of the roles of other workers.
- Communicate nursing ethics to other professions.
- Instil in learners the need to safeguard the individual, family or community when care is endangered by health care personnel.

National Nurses' Associations
- Stimulate co-operation with other related disciplines.
- Develop awareness of ethical issues of other professions.
- Provide guidelines, position statements and discussion fora related to safeguarding people when their care is endangered by health care personnel.

Dissemination of the *ICN Code of Ethics for Nurses*

To be effective, the *Code of Ethics for Nurses* must be familiar to nurses. We encourage you to help with its dissemination to schools of nursing, practising nurses, the nursing press and other mass media. The *Code* should also be disseminated to other health professions, the general public, consumer and policy making groups, and to human rights organisations and employers of nurses.

Glossary of terms used in the *ICN Code of Ethics for Nurses*

Co-operative relationship – A professional relationship based on collegial and reciprocal actions and behaviour that aims to achieve certain goals.

Co-worker – Refers to nurses and other health and non-health related workers and professionals.

Nurse shares with society – A nurse as a health professional and a citizen initiates and supports appropriate action to meet the health and social needs of the public.

Personal health – The mental, physical, social and spiritual well-being of the nurse.

Personal information – Information obtained during a professional contact that is private to an individual or family, and which, when disclosed, may violate the right to privacy, cause inconvenience, embarrassment, or harm to the individual or family.
Related groups – Other nurses, health care workers or other professionals providing service to an individual, family or community and working toward desired goals.

The *ICN Code of Ethics for Nurses* is available at www.icn.ch or by writing to ICN at 3, place Jean-Marteau, CH-1201 Geneva, Switzerland.

THE NMC *CODE OF PROFESSIONAL CONDUCT*

In contrast to the ICN Code, the NMC *Code of Professional Conduct* (2002) is normative (i.e. it is concerned with describing what is done or should be done and seen to be done) and outlines the accountability that follows from the professional responsibility. The underlying values—which are referred to as the values 'of all United Kingdom health care regulatory bodies'—become the headings of the eight clauses. The NMC Code takes it for granted that nurses will have undergone education in professional and nursing ethics, and that they have understood and taken on board these professional values. It is therefore concerned with making clear where the professional boundaries do or should fall. The purpose of the Code is given right at the beginning and there is no doubt: it is to 'inform', as, indeed, would be expected from a regulatory body.

The forerunner of the NMC Code was the UKCC *Code of Professional Conduct for the Nurse, Midwife and Health Visitor*, which was first published in 1983 and revised in 1984 and 1992. The first revisions were made largely from comments that nurses themselves had contributed, having been invited to do so in the first edition of the Code. The third edition (1992) seemed to stem more clearly from the pen of the UKCC itself.

The text of the NMC *Code of Professional Conduct* (2002) is reprinted below with the permission of the Nursing and Midwifery Council.

NURSING AND MIDWIFERY COUNCIL
CODE OF PROFESSIONAL CONDUCT

Protecting the public through professional standards

As a registered nurse or midwife, you are personally accountable for your practice. In caring for patients and clients, you must:

• respect the patient or client as an individual
• obtain consent before you give any treatment or care
• protect confidential information
• co-operate with others in the team
• maintain your professional knowledge and competence
• be trustworthy
• act to identify and minimise risk to patients and clients.

These are the shared values of all the United Kingdom health care regulatory bodies.

This *Code of professional conduct* was published by the Nursing and Midwifery Council in April 2002 and it [came] into effect on 1 June 2002.

1 Introduction

1.1   The purpose of the *Code of professional conduct* is to:
• inform the professions of the standard of professional conduct required of them in the exercise of their professional accountability and practice.
• inform the public, other professions and employers of the standard of professional conduct that they can expect of a registered practitioner.

1.2   As a registered nurse or midwife, you must:
• protect and support the health of individual patients and clients.
• protect and support the health of the wider community.
• act in such a way that justifies the trust and confidence the public have in you.
• uphold and enhance the good reputation of the professions.

1.3 You are personally accountable for your practice. This means that you are answerable for your actions and omissions, regardless of advice or directions from another professional.

1.4 You have a duty of care to your patients and clients, who are entitled to receive safe and competent care.

1.5 You must adhere to the laws of the country in which you are practising.

2 As a registered nurse or midwife, you must respect the patient or client as an individual

2.1 You must recognise and respect the role of patients and clients as partners in their care and the contribution they can make to it. This involves identifying their preferences regarding care and respecting these within the limits of professional practice, existing legislation, resources and the goals of the therapeutic relationship.

2.2 You are personally accountable for ensuring that you promote and protect the interests and dignity of patient and clients, irrespective of gender, age, race, ability, sexuality, economic status, lifestyle, culture and religious or political beliefs.

2.3 You must, at all times, maintain appropriate professional boundaries in the relationships you have with patients and clients. You must ensure that all aspects of the relationship focus exclusively upon the needs of the patient or client.

2.4 You must promote the interests of patients and clients. This includes helping individuals and groups gain access to health and social care, information and support relevant to their needs.

2.5 You must report to a relevant person or authority, at the earliest possible time, any conscientious objection that may be relevant to your professional practice. You must continue to provide care to the best of your ability until alternative arrangements are implemented.

3 As a registered nurse or midwife, you must obtain consent before you give any treatment or care

3.1 All patients and clients have a right to receive information about their condition. You must be sensitive to their needs and respect the wishes of those who refuse or are unable to receive information about their condition. Information should be accurate, truthful and presented in such a way as to make it easily understood. You may need to seek legal or professional advice, or guidance from your employer, in relation to the giving or withholding of consent.

3.2 You must respect patients' and clients' autonomy – their right to decide whether or not to undergo any health care intervention – even where a refusal may result in harm or death to themselves or a foetus, unless a court of law orders to the contrary. This right is protected in law, although in circumstances where the health of the foetus would be severely compromised by any refusal to give consent, it would be appropriate to discuss this matter fully within the team, and possibly to seek external advice and guidance (see clause 4).

3.3 When obtaining valid consent, you must be sure that it is:

- given by a legally competent person
- given voluntarily
- informed.

3.4 You should presume that every patient and client is legally competent unless otherwise assessed by a suitably qualified practitioner. A patient or client who is legally competent can understand and retain treatment information and can use it to make an informed choice.

3.5 Those who are legally competent may give consent in writing, orally or by co-operation. They may also refuse consent. You must ensure that all your discussions and associated decisions relating to obtaining consent are documented in the patient's or client's health care records.

3.6 When patients or clients are no longer legally competent and thus have lost the capacity to consent to or refuse treatment and care, you should try to find out whether they have previously indicated preferences in an advance statement. You must respect any refusal of treatment or care given when they were legally competent, provided that the decision is clearly applicable to the present circumstances and that there is no reason to believe that they have changed their minds. When such a statement is not available, the patients' or clients' wishes, if known, should be taken into account. If these wishes are not known, the criteria for treatment must be that it is in their best interests.

3.7 The principles of obtaining consent apply equally to those people who have a mental illness. Whilst you should be involved in their assessment, it will also be necessary to involve relevant people close to them; this may include a psychiatrist. When patients and clients are detained under statutory powers (mental health acts), you must ensure that you know the circumstances and safeguards needed for providing treatment and care without consent.

3.8 In emergencies where treatment is necessary to preserve life, you may provide care without patients' or clients' consent, if they are unable to give it, provided you can demonstrate that you are acting in their best interests.

3.9 No-one has the right to give consent on behalf of another competent adult. In relation to obtaining consent for a child, the involvement of those with parental responsibility in the consent procedure is usually necessary, but will depend on the age and understanding of the child. If the child is under the age of 16 in England and Wales, 12 in Scotland and 17 in Northern Ireland, you must be aware of legislation and local protocols relating to consent.

3.10 Usually the individual performing a procedure should be the person to obtain the patient's or client's consent. In certain circumstances, you may seek consent on behalf of colleagues if you have been specially trained for that specific area of practice.

3.11 You must ensure that the use of complementary or alternative therapies is safe and in the interests of patients and clients. This must be discussed with the team as part of the therapeutic process and the patient or client must consent to their use.

4 As a registered nurse or midwife, you must co-operate with others in the team

4.1 The team includes the patient or client, the patient's or client's family, informal carers and health and social care professionals in the National Health Service, independent and voluntary sectors.

4.2 You are expected to work co-operatively within teams and to respect the skills, expertise and contributions of your colleagues. You must treat them fairly and without discrimination.

4.3 You must communicate effectively and share your knowledge, skill and expertise with other members of the team as required for the benefit of patients and clients.

4.4 Health care records are a tool of communication within the team. You must ensure that the health care record for the patient or client is an accurate account of treatment, care planning and delivery. It should be consecutive, written with the involvement of the patient or client wherever practicable and completed as soon as possible after an event has occurred. It should provide clear evidence of the care planned, the decisions made, the care delivered and the information shared.

4.5 When working as a member of a team, you remain accountable for your professional conduct, any care you provide and any omission on your part.

4.6 You may be expected to delegate care delivery to others who are not registered nurses or midwives. Such delegation must not compromise existing care but must be directed to meeting the needs and serving the interests of patients and clients. You remain accountable for the appropriateness of the delegation, for ensuring that the person who does the work is able to do it and that adequate supervision or support is provided.

4.7 You have a duty to co-operate with internal and external investigations.

5 As a registered nurse or midwife, you must protect confidential information

5.1 You must treat information about patients and clients as confidential and use it only for the purposes for which it was given. As it is impractical to obtain consent every time you need to share information with others, you should ensure that patients and clients understand that some information may be made available to other members of the team involved in the delivery of care. You must guard against breaches of confidentiality by protecting information from improper disclosure at all times.

5.2 You should seek patients' and clients' wishes regarding the sharing of information with their family and others. When a patient or client is considered incapable of giving permission, you should consult relevant colleagues.

5.3 If you are required to disclose information outside the team that will have personal consequences for patients or clients, you must obtain their consent. If the patient or client withholds consent, or if consent cannot be obtained for whatever reason, disclosures may be made only where:

- they can be justified in the public interest (usually where disclosure is essential to protect the patient or client or someone else from the risk of significant harm)
- they are required by law or by order of a court.

5.4 Where there is an issue of child protection, you must act at all times in accordance with national and local policies.

6 As a registered nurse or midwife, you must maintain your professional knowledge and competence

6.1 You must keep your knowledge and skills up-to-date throughout your working life. In particular, you should take part regularly in learning activities that develop your competence and performance.

6.2 To practise competently, you must possess the knowledge, skills and abilities required for lawful, safe and effective practice without direct supervision. You must acknowledge the limits of your professional competence and only undertake practice and accept responsibilities for those activities in which you are competent.

6.3 If an aspect of practice is beyond your level of competence or outside your area of registration, you must obtain help and supervision from a competent practitioner until you and your employer consider that you have acquired the requisite knowledge and skill.

6.4 You have a duty to facilitate students of nursing and midwifery and others to develop their competence.

6.5 You have a responsibility to deliver care based on current evidence, best practice and, where applicable, validated research when it is available.

7 As a registered nurse or midwife, you must be trustworthy

7.1 You must behave in a way that upholds the reputation of the professions. Behaviour that compromises this reputation may call your registration into question even if [it] is not directly connected to your professional practice.

7.2 You must ensure that your registration status is not used in the promotion of commercial products or services, declare any financial or other interests in relevant organisations providing such goods or services and ensure that your professional judgement is not influenced by any commercial considerations.

7.3 When providing advice regarding any product or service relating to your professional role or area of practice, you must be aware of the risk that, on account of your professional title or qualification, you could be perceived by the patient or client as endorsing the product. You should fully explain the advantages and disadvantages of alternative products so that the patient or client can make an informed choice. Where you recommend a specific product, you must ensure that your advice is based on evidence and is not for your own commercial gain.

7.4 You must refuse any gift, favour or hospitality that might be interpreted, now or in the future, as an attempt to obtain preferential consideration.

7.5 You must neither ask for nor accept loans from patients, clients or their relatives and friends.

8 As a registered nurse or midwife, you must act to identify and minimise the risk to patients and clients

8.1 You must work with other members of the team to promote health care environments that are conducive to safe, therapeutic and ethical practice.

8.2 You must act quickly to protect patients and clients from risk if you have good reason to believe that you or a colleague, from your own or another profession, may not be fit to practise for reasons of conduct, health or competence. You should be aware of the terms of legislation that offer protection for people who raise concerns about health and safety issues.

8.3 Where you cannot remedy circumstances in the environment of care that could jeopardise standards of practice, you must report them to a senior person with sufficient authority to manage them and also, in the case of midwifery, to the supervisor of midwives. This must be supported by a written record.

8.4 When working as a manager, you have a duty toward patients and clients, colleagues, the wider community and the organisation in which you and your colleagues work. When facing professional dilemmas, your first consideration in all activities must be the interests and safety of patients and clients.

8.5 In an emergency, in or outside the work setting, you have a professional duty to provide care. The care provided would be judged against what could reasonably be expected from someone with your knowledge, skills and abilities when placed in those particular circumstances.

Glossary

Accountable   Responsible for something or to someone.

Care   To provide help or comfort.

Competent   Possessing the skills and abilities required for lawful, safe and effective professional practice without direct supervision.

Patient and client   Any individual or group using a health service.

Reasonable   The case of Bolam v Friern Hospital Management Committee (1957) produced the following definition of what is reasonable.
                         "The test is the standard of the ordinary skilled man exercising and professing to have that special skill. A man need not possess the highest expert skill at the risk of being found negligent ... it is sufficient if he exercises the skill of an ordinary man exercising that particular art."
                         This definition is supported and clarified by the case of Bolitho v City and Hackney Health Authority.

Further information

This *Code of professional conduct* is available on the Nursing and Midwifery Council's website at www.nmc-uk.org. Printed copies can be obtained by writing to the Publications Department, Nursing and Midwifery Council, 23 Portland Place, London W1B 1PZ, by fax on 020 7436 2924 or by e-mail at publications@nmc-uk.org. A wide range of NMC standards and guidance publications expand upon and develop many of the professional issues and themes identified in the *Code of professional conduct*. All are available on the NMC's website. A list of current NMC publications is available either on the website or on request from the Publications Department as above.

Enquiries about the issues addressed in the *Code of professional conduct* should be directed in the first instance to the NMC's professional advice service at the address above, by e-mail at advice@nmc-uk.org, by telephone on 020 7333 6541/6550/6553 or by fax on 020 7333 6538.

The Nursing and Midwifery Council will keep this *Code of professional conduct* under review and any comments, suggestions or requests for further clarification are welcome, both from practitioners and members of the public. These should be addressed to the Director of Policy and Standards, NMC, 23 Portland Place, London W1B 1PZ.

April 2002

Summary

- As a registered nurse or midwife, you must respect the patient or client as an individual.
- As a registered nurse or midwife, you must obtain consent before you give any treatment or care.
- As a registered nurse or midwife, you must co-operate with others in the team.
- As a registered nurse or midwife, you must protect confidential information.
- As a registered nurse or midwife, you must maintain your professional knowledge and competence.
- As a registered nurse or midwife, you must be trustworthy.
- As a registered nurse or midwife, you must act to identify and minimise the risk to patients and clients.

Perhaps what is most noticeable about this fourth edition of the Code is its length. From what used to be a small two-page document that could be known by heart, it has now become a text to be reckoned with. From the earlier 16 clauses it has now shrunk to half that number, but subclauses elaborate the main topics. The main points are listed at the beginning and summarised again at the end of the document; they can in fact be memorised quite easily. This is much to be commended. A more detailed discussion of the clauses follows.

1 Introduction

1.1 The much more thorough approach to this Code is visible at the beginning in that its purpose is stated first of all: the Code is here to inform the professions of what is expected of them, and to inform the public what they can expect of practitioners. If each side knows what to expect of the other, there is less ambiguity.

1.2 The interesting phrase here seems to be that nurses and midwives have to 'act in such a way that justifies the trust and confidence the public have in you.' Trust is very easily lost and not readily restored. Trusting someone is as much a personal preference as a basis in fact. Polls have shown that nurses are often more trusted than consultants, but it is not clear what the basis is for this. Trust seems to be earned more than implicitly given. There is something about character operating here, and this is in the realm of morality.

1.3 It seems that a lawyer has studied the text in detail, particularly this subclause, which is good advice. Accountability means 'that you are answerable for your actions and omissions, regardless of advice or directions from another professional.' The Code applies to registered practitioners, but the same advice and standard of care apply to students, who need to be aware that 'inexperience is no defence' (Tschudin and McGregor 2001, p. 59). It is therefore not surprising that subclause 1.5 refers to adhering to the laws of the country in which a practitioner works.

2 As a registered nurse or midwife, you must respect the patient or client as an individual

The individuality of the person is stressed here; this surely means that, as such, the person needs to be given individual attention and is given individualised and holistic care.

2.1 Treating patients and clients as partners in care is the norm, and it may seem even a little patronising to mention this in a code. However, for patients and clients to see this in a code may give them the necessary confidence. There is also the possibility of reminding patients and clients of their own responsibility in care, if necessary.

2.2 This is an interesting list of items against which patients and clients should not be discriminated; it is wider than other similar lists. There seems to be a hint here ('economic status') to guard against the excesses of some of the more blatant means of rationing health care, such as QALYs (see Ch. 4).

2.3 The 'appropriate professional boundaries' of this subclause sound rather cautious when the next sentence urges practitioners to ensure that 'all aspects of the relationship focus exclusively upon the needs of the patient or client'. The patient may perceive a 'need' that could be very demanding, such as requests for frequent counselling, possible sexual favours, or simply attention. The need expressed in the heading, to treat patients and clients as individuals, and this need, may be conflicting; this is where a good basis of personal as well as professional values surely needs to be in place and functioning.

2.5 'Conscientious objection' could be a minefield for practitioners objecting to carrying out various practices that could come under this heading. This is perhaps a good example of how even such a comprehensive code needs to be interpreted in specific situations.

3 As a registered nurse of midwife, you must obtain consent before you give any treatment or care

No less than eleven subclauses make this by far the most comprehensive clause.

3.1 The word 'truthful' is very welcome here. Truth has been very conspicuous by its absence in most nursing and medical codes until very recently.

3.2 This is a clear reference (without mentioning the word) to the practice by members of the Jehovah's Witness Church of not accepting blood transfusions. People of a particular conviction, belief or practice may not be happy with the treatments or interventions offered, and too often they have been made to feel inadequate or even like criminals. This is not compatible with treating individuals; hence it is a welcome elaboration of a basic value in health care.

3.5 Making it clear that consent is more than a signature on a dotted line is an important addition in this Code. The whole notion of consent is expanding, and there will no doubt be many different foci of consent in the future, not least on when consent is needed and what level of involvement is needed by both parties. Refusing consent has often been understood as a rejection of either the person offering treatment or the treatment itself. However, in other situations in life there is not the same pressure to conform; it is important that this is also beginning to be understood in health care.

3.6 The area of advance directives has received much attention in recent years. It is still often stressed that 'living wills' are not legal documents; it is therefore interesting that this subclause promotes them unconditionally. This and other subclauses are thus implying that the views and wishes of families and friends ('clients') are to be heard and respected. What is 'in their best interests', however, will always be contentious and may need help with understanding and interpretation (see also subclause 3.8).

3.7 This subclause refers mainly to care in the mental health field, where treatment is often given without consent and frequently on a compulsory basis. As well as this Code, local guidelines and policies need to be known and followed.

3.9 It is rather strange that within one country there is such wide variation in the age of consent. Part of professional practice is to be familiar with the legal requirements (see also subclause 1.5).

3.11 It is good that complementary and alternative therapies are officially acknowledged in this subclause because they have been used and practised for such a long time.

4 As a registered nurse or midwife, you must cooperate with others in the team

4.4 This subclause is concerned with health care records. These are often of great concern, mainly because of the time they consume in keeping them up to date, and in their accuracy. Writing good records is as much an art as the rest of nursing, and is perhaps something that should be taught in much greater detail during basic nurse education (see also subclause 8.3).

4.6 Although subclause 1.3 makes it clear that everyone is answerable for their own actions and omissions, subclause

4.6 makes it equally clear that a delegated action remains the responsibility of the delegator. Spelling out the various duties and responsibilities is helpful, especially now that other advisory documents previously published by the UKCC are no longer applicable, and this Code replaces and incorporates them. It remains to be seen if this will be a useful subclause.

5 As a registered nurse or midwife, you must protect confidential information

5.1 Like the trust of subclause 1.2, confidentiality is easily lost and not readily restored. There have, however, been debates (Cain 1997, 1998, Wainwright 1998) if nurses can even use patient examples in class discussions for fear of divulging confidential information. Every situation will be different, so it is important to keep the general rule. It is, however, also important to realise that, while all health information about people is essentially confidential, some information is more confidential than other.

6 As a registered nurse or midwife, you must maintain your professional knowledge and competence

This clause seems to be the NMC's own bid to ensure that practitioners stay on the right side of the Council's records of registration.

6.1 This subclause refers implicitly to Post-Registration Education and Practice (known as 'PREP'). The UKCC was for long hailed as an example of professional registration when other similar professions were lagging behind. Keeping up with professional development is not a luxury, but a need. It should therefore also be incumbent on employers to ensure that they give enough weight to their staff's education. Simply demanding it of staff without giving them the possibilities is therefore perhaps a one-sided requirement here.

6.5 The expression 'validated research' is significant here, as it relates to subclause 6.1. There would be much more research available and validated if nurses had enough resources. So often a small gesture of support can go a very long way. Giving the necessary support to carry through some research or change some practice based on research should be part of regular practice, but so is the prior need to support and respect the individual, who in this instance is the nurse or midwife.

8 As a registered nurse or midwife, you must act to identify and minimise the risk to patients and clients

8.2 In the UKCC Code of 1992, clause 13 concerning 'the health or safety of colleagues ... at risk' was often seen as the clause that not only allowed snooping on others, but actually encouraged it. In the new form, the individual 'you' is also included, thus making it a much improved clause, no longer only concerning 'them' only.

8.5 There is no doubt now, that 'once a nurse, always a nurse', and being off-duty cannot be used as an excuse. This is not always a comfortable position, but this Code makes it clear that being a professional does carry a duty to help 'reasonably' in any situation. It is therefore also welcome that the word 'reasonable' is defined in the glossary in the words of the Bolam test.

This is a comprehensive code that will take its place among other similar documents in an increasing number of countries. The previous edition of the UKCC Code lasted for 10 years; this edition has at least that much life in it. For any code to be useful, it must however be regularly updated and amended. Although this is a good document, it is not written in stone. Nurses change, the profession changes and society changes; the present document is valid for now, but another edition will certainly be needed in due course.

DECLARATIONS

Declarations are statements of 'principle, reflecting consensus, shared values, and professional solidarity. They remind practitioners of acknowledged professional obligations but seldom seek to justify positions adopted, these being held as self-evident' (Sommerville 1997, pp. 65–66). Declarations have taken on an air of solemnity, often of urgency, and mostly contain statements of implied rights rather than of conduct. These facts are generally not disputed, but they are nevertheless not easily put into practice everywhere. Among the best known such declarations are:

- The Declaration of Independence of the United States of America was written in 1776. Its second paragraph is of interest here in its choice of words and the order in which they are set: 'All men are created equal ... they are endowed by their Creator with certain inalienable Rights, that among these are Life, Liberty and the pursuit of Happiness.'
- The Universal Declaration of Human Rights was adopted by the United Nations in Paris on 10 December 1948. This Declaration has 30 articles, outlining the 'inherent dignity and the equal and inalienable rights of all members of the human family [which] is the foundation of freedom, justice and peace in the world'. This Declaration led to the Convention for the Protection of Human Rights and Fundamental Freedoms (the European Convention on Human Rights) in 1950. This in turn led to the (UK) Human Rights Act of 1998.

The World Medical Association has issued many declarations. These documents are binding on doctors, but are mentioned here because in certain circumstances nurses are implied because of their close cooperation with doctors. A selection of these declarations contains the Declaration of Helsinki (1964, revised several times, the latest in 2000). This document is 'a statement of ethical principles to provide guidance to physicians and other participants in medical research involving human subjects' (World Health Organization 2001). The Declaration of Sydney (1968), is a statement on the determination of death. The Declaration of Oslo (1970), a statement on therapeutic abortion, has as its last clause the following: 'This statement, while it is endorsed by the General Assembly of the World Medical Association, is not to be regarded as binding on any individual member association unless it is adopted by that member association' (Duncan et al 1981).

The Declaration of Tokyo was adopted in 1975. This document

contains guidelines for doctors 'concerning torture and other cruel, inhuman or degrading treatment or punishment' in relation to detention and imprisonment. Willingly or unwillingly, nurses may be in situations of assisting doctors in dubious 'research' or procedures that may be covered by this declaration.

Many declarations are updated when new material makes the text less relevant. There is often fierce debate around certain subjects, as was the case surrounding the wording of the 2000 amendment of the Declaration of Helsinki.

Other bodies also issue declarations, such as UNESCO, which produced The Universal Declaration on the Human Genome and Human Rights in 1997.

The ICN issues many position statements and notices, often in response to world events, such as wars and conflict, or to specific situations, such as well-reported executions. Position statements are also regularly updated. Indeed, the ICN has taken an increasingly vocal stance on human rights and disseminates the statements widely. It also uses press statements because they can have a wider circulation and a quicker impact. The ICN often combines with other relevant bodies in making joint statements. A good example is the statement issued by the ICN, the World Health Professions Association and the International Pharmaceutical Federation on 7 January 2002, which jointly condemns human cloning. This followed earlier media reports that the practice has been attempted. All ICN texts are available on the ICN website at: www.icn.org

Most of the declarations available are concerned with human rights. Precisely what human rights are is not always very clear. Shashi Tharoor (2001, p. 34–35) has argued that human rights 'derive from the mere fact of being human'. He considers the influence of philosophy, culture, the north/south arguments, and religion to have distorted the real value of human rights. Declarations about human or universal rights have generally been made by western cultures and concern western ideals, in particular concepts such as individuality and nationhood. Cultures change and are not homogeneous, and the individual is not necessarily the most important person. Tharoor writes, '[I]n Africa it is usually the community that protects and nurtures the individual: "I am because we are, and because we are, therefore I am".' Women's rights cannot be universal 'when in some societies marriage is seen not as a contract between two individuals but as an alliance between lineages'. It is only 'the availability of political and civil rights which give people the opportunity to draw attention to their needs and to demand action from the government'. For states simply not to interfere with individual freedoms is not enough when there are millions of people around the globe who are hungry, deprived, illiterate and jobless. Tharoor says that 'human rights ... start with breakfast'. In his view, human rights should reflect our common humanity with its diversity, and not fundamentally contradict the ideals and aspirations of any society. This may be a tall order because powerful states and institutions (e.g. the USA and the International Monetary Fund) want to ensure that people and nations conform to the ideals and sanctions imposed or created by the institutions. Perhaps it is useful that human rights are not fixed entities, and that in fact respect and attention for individuals and situations are increasingly challenged and considered to be essential.

With the passing of the Human Rights Act, 1998, into UK law, people as a whole have become more aware of their rights and duties. At the time of writing it is too early to say how much nurses may have to be made more aware of this Act for their daily work. Education for human rights is, however, an increasingly urgent topic (Chamberlain 2001).

Declarations and codes are useful in that they provide generalised guidelines. They have their limitations, particularly when specific issues are tested against them. The nursing codes direct; they do not protect. They stimulate thinking but they do not provide walls within which it is safe to act. In the overall scheme of an ethic of caring they state perhaps the obvious, or the implied, but they also sharpen the perception of care.

6

Rights and responsibilities

RIGHT VERSUS RESPONSIBILITY

An ethic of care is based on a relationship. Within this, it is based on the ability to receive through listening, on sharing because those concerned have been heard, and on the ability to respond. If people are to be and remain creative, they have to respond to others and events around them. This gives them the ability to care. Responsibility comes with caring and leads to caring.

Precisely what rights are, and how we claim them, is not easily stated. Our basic human rights exist simply because we are human. The state makes it a duty to protect its individual citizens by providing basic goods and services, such as clean water, food and shelter. The state also provides certain legal rights, such as the right to vote, and the right to be protected and defended. A system of policing, and of civil and criminal law, are in force to maintain these rights. To claim any right, someone has to have a responsibility to fulfil that right.

Rights have become important because the basic relationships between nurse and patient, doctor and patient, institution and patient, and state and individual have been abused too often in paternalistic guises and forms. An abuse of power results in a loss of responsibility and degrades not only individuals but also societies. Thus, Anne Davis and her colleagues (1997) state that: 'Legally, a right has to do with the power of an individual to change something or to keep it the same, such as a contractual relationship for health care benefits in a managed care organization' (p. 85). The right to health care means that some organisation or institution (or the state, as in the UK) has the responsibility to supply the health care. However, citizens have the responsibility to pay their taxes to fund the care. Newer rights, such as the right to have a child or the right to die, are much more disputed. Are these 'real' rights and who has the responsibility to supply them? All ethical issues are mainly 'boundary issues' between the known and the unknown, so these issues have been debated a great deal in recent years, often with very conflicting opinions.

For the present purpose, rights and responsibilities can be considered at five levels:

- personal rights and responsibilities
- nurses' rights and responsibilities
- patients' rights and responsibilities
- institutional rights and responsibilities
- societal rights and responsibilities.

PERSONAL RIGHTS AND RESPONSIBILITIES

Rights derive from respect for the person within a social context. As such, therefore, rights need to be seen within a wider context. However, we also use the word 'right' for quite personal aspects of living. We have the right to live the lifestyle that suits us best. We have a right to bring up our children as we think fit. We have rights to associate with the people we choose. These issues concern mostly some notion of privacy; we are left in peace to get on with our own lives. All this, however, is stated only in contrast to some social context. We have the right to live our lives as it suits us, as long as it fits in with the people around us who may depend on us. We can bring up our children as we like, as long as it does not harm them. Consenting adults have the right to engage in unusual activities, if other people are not affected. The difficulty is that, in most instances, other people are affected: neighbours are disturbed; children suffer; and people may have to be rescued, or they may become ill as a result of unusual activities. This means that the state has to pick up the pieces from people's 'rights'. Thiroux's (1995) principle of individual freedom accords with the idea of privacy outlined here. Such a principle of individual freedom is possible only within a context of the other principles; that is, doing good, being honest and pursuing justice also have to be considered. Individual rights are also shared rights.

Being responsible

The concept of responsibility can be divided into the more personal aspect of being responsible, and the more legal aspect of having responsibility (discussed below).

Being responsible grows out of being engaged with people. It also grows out of values that come to be important as persons take their stand fully in the world. We learn this perhaps first because of the inner bond created with our children (van Hooft 1995). Being responsible is altruistic, but it is also more than just 'doing good'. It is actively taking a part and an interest in a cause. This may be a job, or charitable work, or local or national government. A person who feels involved is a person who is responsible.

Being responsible does not mean bearing everybody's burdens. That would exclude the aspect of reciprocity.

To be responsible is a truly ethical act: being aware of what is happening (descriptive ethics), and prepared to engage with it and work for its positive advance (normative ethics) in society. James Robertson (1998) speaks of 'the right to be responsible' (p. 72).

Having responsibility

To have responsibility means to be answerable to someone or something specific, usually defined by contract. This is normally also a job for which the person is paid.

A contract lays down what the parameters of the job are, and the job holder acts within these limits. Responsibility here means to use all one's powers to the limits, not just some of them. It means also to know the boundaries clearly and to be accountable, especially if any limits have been overstepped. It would be irresponsible of a student nurse on her or his first placement to catheterise a patient. It would be equally irresponsible for a ward manager to see a patient with symptoms of fluid retention and do nothing about it, but a student nurse may not yet be able to recognise the symptoms.

Nurses are constantly asked to perform duties for which they may not have been trained, or do so of their own volition. Most of these extend either into the other professions' realms. The Nursing and Midwifery Council (NMC) Code (2002) is specific about such situations: 'you must possess the knowledge, skills and abilities required for lawful, safe and effective practice without direct supervision' (clause 6.2). This is not only to safeguard nurses but also patients, who have the right to receive care from those who are trained and educated to give that particular care. 'Having responsibility' equates with professional accountability. Andrew Edgar (1994) states that 'the practitioner can look to no one else to take the blame for failures' (p. 156). Although this is put negatively, Robertson (1998) believes that the establishment of many new rights has actually diminished our rights to take responsibility for ourselves. However, as 'the institutions of modern society, such as the national labour market, become less able to deliver the goods we require of them, such as jobs, we shall find it necessary to take more responsibility for ourselves' (p. 72). This is seen here in the context of finding jobs for ourselves, but it is also clear that within our jobs we take new responsibilities for ourselves. Within nursing this is expressed in many examples of nurse specialists, nurse practitioners and nurse consultants. The professional issues themselves are addressed in Chapter 9. Here they are mentioned in relation to rights and responsibilities. These jobs and aspects of professional work do indeed give nurses 'the right to be responsible'. There is no doubt that people who have responsibility for certain areas of work or life, are more engaged in their work or life and feel more satisfied because their creative capacities are addressed and used.

NURSES' RIGHTS AND RESPONSIBILITIES

The nurses' rights are the employer's duties. The patients' rights are the nurses' duties.

Nurses' contracts give them the right to an established salary, paid without fail, specified numbers of days or weeks of holiday, and the right to sick leave. In return, their duty is to give care to the level of their training, education and position, without fail, or to inform the relevant authority when this cannot be done.

Nurses have the right to work in a healthy environment, free from danger of accidents to themselves or other health hazards. Many trusts and health employers also display notices on premises that all personnel have the right to work free from fear of attack or harassment. It is the duty of the employing authority to supply these conditions.

Nurses should be able to work in an environment that is also psychologically, emotionally and spiritually healthy. This depends on relationships with other staff so that an atmosphere is created that is conducive to work and good health, and is supportive of staff.

It is important at all levels that staff generally, and nurses in particular, are able to exercise their professional judgement. Nurses who are hemmed in by layers of hierarchy and mountains of policies cannot make independent decisions. Thus, a right that nurses have is to be as free of bureaucracy as possible. This freedom does not lead to bad practice as is often feared, but rather to more responsible action, because the person is trusted. Flatter organisational structures and support rather than sanctions are two conditions that enable nurses to develop personally and professionally.

The basic duty or responsibility of nurses is to care. This is seen most clearly in their relationship with patients. If patients are to be in a well-cared-for environment, then nurses have to care about that environment. This includes equipment, adequate buildings, cleanliness, and regular supplies. Allowing ward and departmental managers and leaders to be budget holders will greatly contribute to this, but it should not lead to nurses spending hours on the telephone calling all the agencies for the best nurse, or having to search the web for who has the cheapest light bulb in the country. Linda Aiken (1998) wrote simply: 'if you give nurses control or autonomy they can deliver much better care than if they are told what to do ... They just need to be given the authority' (p. 31).

The human rights organisation Amnesty International (1997) has published a document detailing human rights violations against nurses. Although this may be far from most nurses' experience, it is one aspect of the international aspect of nursing that affects all practitioners. Nurses have increasing contact with colleagues in far-flung parts of the world, and may meet nurses as refugees or asylum seekers who have been subjected to corporal punishment, forensic investigations or imprisonment. Amnesty International 'believes that nurses and nursing organisations have an important role to play in the defence of human rights in general and the protection of nurses' rights in particular' (cover blurb).

When the emphasis is on basic human rights and the ethical stance is on respecting the person and believing that 'people matter', rights and responsibilities are not hedged with claims and counterclaims. The duty to care well for patients may therefore become again 'the right to be responsible'.

PATIENTS' RIGHTS AND RESPONSIBILITIES

The UK's *Patient's Charter* came into effect in April 1992 (Department of Health 1992), when it was hailed as a ground-breaking document. Very soon, however, health personnel realised that one of its main shortcomings was that it does not make clear who has the responsibility to fulfil the rights mentioned there. Patients were claiming their right to wait no more than 20 minutes in outpatient departments, but no one was responsible for implementing this right. It became clear that this was a one-sided document because the NHS could not claim anything from patients in the way of responsibility, such as making sure that they cancel appointments rather than simply not turn up. The Department of Health published the sequel, *The Patient's Charter and You*, in 1995 (Department of Health 1995), listing some of the ways in which patients can help the NHS. However, this document has not had the same impact as the original Patient's Charter, and both are now largely sidelined by charters produced by local trusts or health employers.

Informed consent has often been seen as the process by which patients agree to care and treatments; being informed meant that they would therefore cooperate. Increasingly, it has also come to be understood that informing patients does give them the necessary tools *not* to agree to the care or treatments proposed. They have the right to say 'no', and do so in an informed way and without fear of pressure or sanction.

For many years the main area where patients exercised their right not to have certain treatments was in the care of Jehovah's Witnesses who refuse blood transfusions. However, this issue has forced to the fore other aspects of care that concern patients' rights:

- This debate and the ethical stance taken has contributed to the need to pay more attention to individual differences and to respect the rights of minority populations for adequate cultural and religious care.
- It has also forced physicians and scientists to consider other therapies for certain diseases and disabilities.
- The individual's determination becomes a limit to the physician's actions and the 'therapeutic privilege' that doctors claim must benefit the patient's life.

- Patients may not be as autonomous as has often been taken for granted, but families' and communities' decisions and influence need to play the role accorded to them by patients (J Washburn, personal communication 2000).

Patients have rights not to wait for more than certain set times for operations, for appointments, or for an emergency ambulance to arrive. These issues would be taken for granted in a private organisation. Not-for-profit services, however, can never be run quite on the same principles as private institutions because their emphasis is different. Patients therefore need to be protected against misuse of their rights and their humanity.

Clearly, the main right that patients have is to be treated according to their needs. The intensified debate within the NHS has therefore been to define 'needs'. Various institutions, such as the National Institute for Clinical Excellence, the Commission for Health Improvement, and the National Patient Safety Agency, function to regulate the different aspects of care and need. Patients have the right not to be harmed. This includes issues of infection such as methicillin-resistant *Staphylococcus aureus*, HIV, and hepatitis B and C from infected blood. It also includes issues in midwifery practice and all other areas where nurses are employed, such as GP surgeries, clinics, schools and industry.

According to Douglas Olsen (2000), patients have their own responsibility for optimum health care. Two types of choices lead to health problems: life-style and non-compliance. However, Olsen argues that physicians should not decide on patients' life-style choices, but that this is society's role, leading to setting prospective consequences in the form of taxes, education and prevention.

The various aspects of citizen responsibility already mentioned apply at all levels of patient responsibility: respecting each other as persons, and respecting each other's time and resources. This includes such common courtesies, such as cancelling appointments when they are not needed, returning equipment, and not attacking staff verbally or physically. Living in an age where we can have most of what we want now can lead to the impression that we can also have health now, attention now, and satisfaction now. Unfortunately we tend then to forget that this depends on people, not on machines, and people do not act like machines.

INSTITUTIONAL RIGHTS AND RESPONSIBILITIES

Customers' rights are the institution's duties. Patients and personnel must have certain expectations that can be assured.

A trust or other health employer as an institution has first of all a duty to care for its patients. It takes this from the state, which sees health care for all as its duty and as the individual citizen's right. As such it is merely carrying out its legal responsibility. This is a contractual relationship, so the relationship with employers is not always easy, tending to be one of suspicion and calculated friendliness.

Ethics is above law, so a good action is only good if there is a sense of 'excellence' attached to it. An institution, therefore, acts ethically if it prevents, foresees, actualises potential and humanises. It sees its duties not only as strictly 'having to', but more as 'wanting to'. Such institutions ensure that contracts are maintained, and that buildings and equipment are serviced regularly and kept in good working order. It means also that staff facilities, such as crèches and car parking are available, and that flexible working hours and contracts are made possible. These things sound 'obvious', but it is a fact that institutions look after themselves first of all, only secondarily looking after their employees and members of the public.

The rights of an institution are that it needs to expect its employees to respect policies, bylaws and measures that ensure good working conditions, and also help others to respect them.

An inherent difficulty with all institutions is that negative rights tend to be emphasised (i.e. the protection of what we have) rather than the positive rights (i.e. the provision of what we need). Individual and collective rights and duties are liable to conflict with each other because what an individual needs (such as health care) cannot be provided by the collective membership. The concept of advocacy arose out of such situations.

The ethical principles mostly involved here are those of justice and fairness, and non-maleficence (see Ch. 4). It is difficult to say, however, that any one aspect of ethics is more important than another, because all principles and approaches are equally necessary. All the same, justice in health care is increasingly of concern, with ever greater and more needs, largely because of an ageing population and decreasing resources.

SOCIETAL RIGHTS AND RESPONSIBILITIES

Much has been said and written in recent years about society and its decline, needs, hopes and possibilities. Issues such as global warming, climate changes and the state of the world's poor nations are never out of public consciousness. Increasing numbers of people see their personal responsibilities also in terms of social and societal responsibilities. What were once considered personal failings or shortcomings are now frequently seen within a wider social setting. Thus, a nurse who makes a drug error is not the only person to blame for the error; the system that allowed or enabled such a mistake to happen is as much to blame. Every system works within other systems and although we may be able to influence one or two systems around us, we are often frustrated by the slowness and inefficiency of other systems that also affect us.

The values held by societies will guide what our rights and responsibilities are. Perhaps too often at the moment, only those who make the loudest noise get what they want. This has frequently been seen in situations where a child has needed an organ transplant or other treatment. When the issue became national news, something happened to resolve it. Martin Melville (1997) considered, that for effective participation, people need 'choice, voice and control' (p. 339). The problem is that there will always be those who are excluded from 'participation' on various grounds that often cannot be foreseen. Many of our small and large systems are geared to exclusion, so when organisations such as the NHS advocate values of inclusion it can therefore be quite problematic. Robertson (1998) asks some pertinent questions that are not out of place here:

What kind of society, and what kind of world, do we want? Do we want a society that fosters self-reliance and equality, or one that reinforces dependency? In deciding what to do or whether a particular initiative is a good one, it still is not generally accepted that the touchstone is: How can the people involved in this problem acquire the capacity to deal with it for themselves? Will this initiative empower all the people affected by it to become more self-reliant? (p. 191).

In considering what rights and duties societies have, especially in the area of health care, these questions (or similar ones) need to be considered. We are not isolated individuals, but all dependent on each other.

- A right claimed by one person is another's responsibility. A right claimed by one person may be another person's right denied. In a situation of scarce resources, one child's transplant gained through media pressure may be another child's transplant denied.
- Who decides which child has more claims?

Nurses need to concern themselves with these questions, locally and nationally. They are at the sharp end of care and practice, and such issues affect them. These may indeed be the nurses' right to be responsible.

7

Making ethical decisions

DECISIONS, DECISIONS ...

Nurses are constantly in situations where decisions have to be made. Many of these are managerial decisions, some are professional decisions, and a number will clearly be ethical decisions. Nurses also have to help patients, clients and colleagues to make decisions.

Ethical decision making is essentially no different from making any other decision. It may feel more difficult to make ethical decisions because ethics as such is a subject that is still rather unclear and has perhaps an aura of a higher level of reasoning being involved. However, ethics is not something intellectual and complicated; it is something everyday and practical. Clearly, there are sometimes major decisions to be made in life, but these are already based on others taken before, and all stem from a background of values, beliefs and attitudes held by the individuals concerned.

Katharine Smith (1996) cites personal and professional characteristics that contribute to ethical decision making. She lists 'thoughts, values, beliefs, ethical principles and moral reasoning, religion, knowledge, experience, conscience, emotions, and relationships with the patient and family (such as trust and rapport)' (p. 20). Smith considered that there are two interrelated and inseparable elements that come into play when ethical decisions have to be made: deliberation and integration. Deliberation is the 'conversation in the head' and actions taken when any decision has to be made; integration is the 'incorporation of the nurse's ethical decision into the clinical context in which it occurs. It includes role, communication patterns, authority and relationships' (p. 21). When these two aspects have been taken care of, then the decision taken and the action carried out are those that are in the patient's best interest.

In a unique study, Arie van der Arend and Corine Remmers-van den Hurk (1999) detailed the kinds of problems Dutch nurses consider to be of an ethical nature. The study considered also the seriousness of the problems described and how these varied between the different care settings in which the study was done. Right across the spectrum, nurses considered that problems with the organisation were the most serious, and problems with other disciplines generally ranked highly. They were considered as moral problems most often in situations in which the nurses felt powerless because nothing more could be done for the patient; the patient was suffering because of slow transfer arrangements to other care facilities; institutional rules obstructed nursing care; and the privacy of patients and their families was insufficiently facilitated or guaranteed. The authors found that the less influence nurses considered they had in such situations, the more they experienced them as moral problems.

In most decision making situations it is necessary to consider how problems arise, what they are, and what can be done about them.

MORAL PROBLEMS

When is a problem a moral or ethical problem and when is it not? There may be clear situations, such as when trying to cover up a mistake or when going against one's conscience or 'better judgement', or when having to decide if a patient should be moved to another department. The first is possibly a moral or ethical problem, but the second is more likely a professional or managerial decision. Both situations have to do with values, motives, experience, and weighing up possible personal and professional outcomes.

van der Arend and Remmers-van den Hurk (1999) detailed the moral problems they found in their survey. They are too many to mention, but their four broad problem areas cover the following situations:

- Synchronising actions and policies, for example:
  —powerlessness that nothing can be done
  —rules obstructing 'measured care'
  —commercialisation of care or means
  —disagreement with prescribed actions
  —unclear resuscitation rules

- Actions of colleagues, for example:
  —verbal aggressiveness towards patients
  —keeping silent about errors
  —not acting decisively because of fear
  —sedating patients for staff convenience
  —ignoring patients' beliefs
- Actions of physicians in diagnostics and/or treatment:
  —(non-)treatment against patient's wishes
  —painful actions/treatments
  —refusal to come, in spite of necessity
  —tests on people who are dying
  —administering drugs without patients' knowledge
  —withholding food/fluid to encourage death
- Actions of patients or family:
  —taking insufficient responsibility for patients' recovery
  —persuading patients to cooperate
  —family intervening inappropriately
  —being confronted with patients' sexual needs
  —disagreeing with patients' choices.

If a similar survey were to be carried out in the UK, similar results would likely be obtained. In a study carried out in Korea among student nurses, the main problem encountered was disregard of the ethical principle of the value of life by families of patients (Han and Ahn 2000). This meant that family members 'gave up' on their relatives who were dying, not visiting them and not being concerned for them. This may mean that patients are neglected. Although this concern arose in a different culture and health care system from the UK, with increasing cultural diversity all nurses will be meeting with situations that may be somewhat unfamiliar. They therefore have to pay special attention to the needs, attitudes and sensibilities of people from different ethnic groups.

A distinction needs to be made between a problem and a dilemma. Generally speaking, a dilemma has only two (or more) equally unsatisfactory possibilities. A problem, however, can be solved. Dilemmas will be dealt with in Chapter 8; problems and problem solving in ethical matters are discussed below.

A process of decision making is helpful in moving situations forward by considering how a dilemma can be turned into a problem.

MODELS FOR DECISION MAKING

Ethical decision making is a process like any other decision making, but there may be more elements involved, which may need more reflection and discussion than other decision-making processes. Very often in situations of ethical challenge the nub or central concern is not obvious, or at least not immediately so. Situations develop, and with them also the main focus. The truth emerges, rather than being the starting point.

There have been many attempts made at finding the best or most useful model for decision making. Models *can* be helpful, but they can also be unhelpful. The four principles of bioethics (see Ch. 4) were meant to be the ideal model for ethical decision making, but they have proved to be too restrictive in a climate where diversity is more valued than certainty. Nevertheless, ethical principles need to be considered in decision making, and models for ethical decision making are outlined here. Neither models nor principles should be used exclusively or adhered to slavishly. Models are perhaps most useful in reflection on decisions made, and when learning how and why a particular decision was made or was useful.

Anne Davis and colleagues (1997, p. 47) have established a model consisting of ten elements that can 'assist with the discussion, analysis, and development of ethically supportable decisions'. This model can also be 'adapted for use at the policy development or evaluation level' and used for decisions related to individual patient care. It consists of topics that have to be taken into account, such as 'Identification of the parties or stakeholders involved in the situation or affected by the decision(s) that is made'.

Mary Greipp (1995) 'has designed a model of ethical decision-making to examine those experiences, beliefs and biases that affect reactions to situations and other people' (p. 212). This model needs visual presentation and is recommended for its 'sociological perspective and the global presentation of the interactions between patients and nurses, and those multifactors than can enhance or inhibit the ethical decision-making process'.

Husted's Formal Ethical Decision Making Model (Husted and Husted 1991, p. xi) has as its basis the 'nurse/patient agreement', which the authors describe as necessary for the nurse to be aware of the patient's unique nature. The model is based on six noncontroversial but crucial points, which are: autonomy, veracity, beneficence, freedom, privacy and fidelity.

Ian Thompson and colleagues (2000, pp. 280-281) have outlined a model based on the acronym DECIDE:

D Define the problem(s)
E Ethical review
C Consider the options
I Investigate outcomes
D Decide on action
E Evaluate the results.

This model is graphically illustrated as a circle, with the starting point (the crisis situation) that has to be defined in the middle, and with the next problem to be specified on the horizon. This model is useful because it may be easy to remember a word like 'DECIDE'.

Megan-Jane Johnstone (1994, p. 183) has also designed a model for moral decision making, comprising five steps:

• assessing the situation
• diagnosing or identifying the moral problems
• setting moral goals and planning an appropriate moral course of action
• implementing the moral plan of action
• evaluating the moral outcomes of the action implemented.

All these models have in common a process of moving from the present problematic to a future more satisfactory situation. If there are five or ten intervening steps, this is not so crucial as the fact that they are helpful guides in addressing the necessary points. The main feature of models for ethical (or moral) decision making is that the ethical issues are addressed. It is therefore useful to have at least one point in the model that makes specific reference to what these may be (or reminds users of the model).

A basic model of problem solving is used here rather than any one particular model. Questions from different sources or theories are listed under each of the steps to stimulate further questions and probing. The problem-solving approach may be too linear or even rigid for some readers. It is to be hoped, therefore, that the questions will be sufficiently diverse to make it clear that, in every situation, aspect, problem or reflection there is more to it than that. Milton Mayeroff (1972, p. 9) believes that to care for someone we must know many things. This shows clearly that: (a) caring is more than simply meaning well and carrying out tasks, but needs thorough training and education; and (b) to care ethically for someone needs a relationship in which this knowledge of the other is important.

STEP ONE: WHAT IS HAPPENING? (ASSESSMENT)

Often, a problem is not stated clearly, or, if more than one person is concerned, assumptions are made by all parties that they all know what is going on. All the people concerned will come from different backgrounds, which will mean they have different perceptions and different values. Sometimes a problem is acknowledged only generally, not in detail. 'The care in this trust is not good enough' has to be made into a specific problem before it can be changed. Stating the problem in terms of people is perhaps the most realistic because, eventually, choices and outcomes directly affect people. People matter; every person in every situation matters. It is also worth remembering that all decisions are made within a context or social setting; every decision affects someone else.

The first step essentially asks Niebuhr's main question: 'What is happening?' In an ethic of care this must always be the question of most concern. This is not just curiosity; it shows genuine empathy and a willingness to 'be there', to receive, to share, and to respond with all the compassion, competence, confidence, conscience and commitment possible. Although the question has to be asked, the answer has to be waited for and heard. It may be a short question, but the answer may be very long.

This first step asks questions, gathers information, assesses, and builds up a body of knowledge. It clarifies details, seeing everything in terms of facts. The questions below are not exclusive. They may not be the right ones, and may certainly not be all that need to be asked. They give, however, an idea of the kind of questions that may be necessary or helpful.

- What is happening?
- Who are the people directly involved here?
- Who are the people indirectly involved?
- What is the role of each involved person?

- What is the history of the problem?
- How does each person perceive the problem?
- Who are the key people?
- What are the key people's overall nursing, medical and social situations?
- Is it an actual or a potential problem?
- Why is it a problem that cannot be solved easily?
- Which facts are important? Which facts are irrelevant or unimportant?
- How is this problem like or unlike other situations or similar cases?
- What are the dominant presenting feelings or memories?
- What particular values are involved? Can they be named precisely?
- Is it a question of opposing values?
- Are there any aspects that enhance or go against the conscience of any person involved?
- What are the basic (human) needs involved?
- What are the wants and desires of the individuals concerned?
- How do the needs and wants compare?
- Are there aspects that can be changed or cannot be changed?
- Precisely what are they? Is it possible to list them?
- Is it a question of personal relationships?
- Is it a question of professional relationships?
- Is the futility of further treatment questioned?
- What other relevant considerations are there?

The specifically ethical aspects may need to be considered:

- Is there a clear duty involved for anyone?
- Does this change or influence the situation?
- Is any clause in the code of professional conduct invoked?
- Is it a question of disregarding a specific principle? (Thiroux's (1995) set of principles are used here in preference over other principles.)
- Is the principle of the value of life involved? (i.e. Is it an issue of shortening or prolonging life, questioning the quality of life or the sanctity of life?) Is one person's life dominant in this scenario? Why? In what way?
- What is good or right about the situation; what is not good or right? Who is good or not good; what is right, or not right?
- Is it a problem that should be seen in terms of justice? What is

questioned about justice? Does it concern resources? Which resources?

- Are all persons respected equally?
- Is it a problem of truth telling or honesty, or lack or disregard of it?
- Is it a problem of individual freedom or autonomy?

When all the fact-finding questions have been asked and answered as well as possible, what emerges is a story that needed to be heard. The story becomes the focus and ethical decisions can be made with it, in conjunction with it, and from within it. In an ethic of care it matters that relationships, receptivity and responsiveness are valued. The following questions are therefore also necessary:

- Has everybody said all they needed to say?
- Does everybody feel they have been heard well enough?
- Has anything relevant not been said yet?
- What may be the possible blind spots?
- How have relationships been affected by this problem?
- Which are the significant relationships involved?
- What do any 'significant others' say, feel, convey or wish to happen?
- How does that affect the other relationships?
- Who has suffered, and in what way, so far?
- What are the main feelings expressed by the various parties?
- What do they indicate, or point to?
- How has care been affected so far?

An ethic of care will endeavour to see as many points as possible. This will involve in particular any relationships with friends, families, the wider community, and any other contexts, such as groups or societies involved or respected. Each is important, each needs to be respected. Only when everyone and everything is respected can the story begin to make sense and move towards a 'fitting answer'.

STEP TWO: WHAT WOULD HAPPEN IF...? (PLANNING)

Step two, the planning stage, looks towards the future. Standing in the present, the people involved can speculate what the outcomes may be, what possible situations or contexts may be affected and how, and how people's lives may be changed by any decision taken. This is the case whether it is a small or simple decision or a major one. Even how to answer a telephone call may involve some ethical reasoning and behaviour because all our actions have consequences.

- What would happen if...?
- Is it a question of deontology? (i.e. What ought to be done? What would happen if we considered only our duty?)
- Is it a question of teleology? (i.e. Does the outcome or do the consequences matter specifically?)
- Is it a question of responding to the individual, and how all protagonists can be most creative, responsive persons in, through and beyond this situation?

The 'fitting answer' has to be reached; therefore some questions relevant to attaining this goal may be:

- What actions are possible?
- What alternatives are available?
- What alternatives may be possible?
- What are the short-term or long-term possibilities?
- What are the possible outcomes of each action?
- Who will be helped in particular?
- How likely is any one outcome?
- Who will be particularly helped by any one decision?
- Will anybody be hurt by any particular outcome? If so, who and how?
- Will one decision solve the problem, or are further decisions likely to be taken?
- What impact could a decision have on the people involved outside the close circle?
- What factors could militate against a consensus?
- Who else should be consulted?
- Is any other person who should be consulted ready to take part in a decision-making process?
- Will there be an impact on the institution or on society by any one decision?
- Is there a time limit?

According to Jameton (1984), this is the point when ethical theories and principles will now have to be thought through, not only stated, and the problem tested against them. The following questions relate to the principles described by Thiroux (1995):

- In what respect does the principle of the value of life give direction at this stage? The summary of that principle is: 'Human beings should revere life and accept death' (p. 180). In what way should life be revered here (if it is not) or death accepted (if it is not)? Is there an action that has to be taken to uphold this principle, an outcome to be hoped for, or ways looked for by which all involved can be more creative persons?
- In which way is good or right compromised? Can all persons involved be 'good' (i.e. act according to values and conscience, beliefs, principles, moral reasoning, religion, experience and relationships, enhancing the common good, keeping and enhancing integrity, creativity and any other human characteristics that increase rather than decrease personal and societal well-being)?
- How are any specifically planned actions right or wrong for any individual, all those concerned in the situation, and/or the wider context? Will an action affect one or many people, and is that as it should be? How could an action be made more right, more specific and with better consequences?
- What aspects of justice or fairness are involved? (The emphasis here is on distributive justice or equity, not legal justice.) How are justice and equity served by this action? How could justice be harmed by this action? For people to be good, they need to be free, creative and respectful of others not only in thought but also in action. How can justice be seen to be done?
- How is the principle of truth telling or honesty involved? Can all speak the truth freely? Do all of them speak the truth freely? Truth telling enhances relationships; how are the present relationships enhanced by truth or destroyed by untruth? In relationships people become creative and responsive; in what way does truth help them in this fundamental quest to be and become authentic human beings? Is the act of telling the truth itself right, or what would the consequences be if it were, or were not, told? Who may need to speak 'the truth' or how can honesty be enhanced?

- Individual freedom and autonomy are the elements that make human beings unique. Is this principle upheld, or not, by this action? Is coercion evident anywhere? Who gives freedom to whom? Who or what takes freedom from whom or from what?
- Is harm being caused? How can it be minimised?
- Is the general tone of the discussion or search for a solution respectful and conducive to good and right above the merely necessary?

Considering specifically the theories of ethics, some of the questions to be asked should therefore be, does the proposed action or intervention bring:

- An increase of individual good?
- An increase of self-good?
- An increase of the good of a particular group?
- An increase of social good?

An ethic of care considers many other aspects and principles than the traditional ones. Some principles may emerge only as the story is told and heard. Some questions relating specifically to other approaches to ethics may therefore be:

- What is the aim of the story being told here?
- Who or what are the important relationships? Some people consider their pets to be the most important 'person' in their lives.
- What is the fundamental element that cannot be changed?
- What is necessary or desirable for the person concerned to retain her or his integrity? Can it be granted? On what basis?
- Is it a question of habit or maybe cultural belonging that needs to be respected? If it is, why has it not been considered before? What needs to be changed so that it can be respected?
- If there is shame or guilt involved, how can the person be helped or supported to deal with it?
- How can virtues such as courage, honesty, loyalty, humility, fidelity etc. be fostered and practised if they have been considered to be lacking?

The specifically caring side of ethics has one very important question at this step:

- What is the meaning of it?

Viktor Frankl (1962) was very clear that people who have or follow a meaning in their lives are people with a purpose. They strive towards a goal. By doing this their actions are purposeful and are subject to that goal. An ethic of care is conducive to the common good and to 'social solidarity'. Every ethical decision has consequences and people have to live with them. If these consequences can be seen not in terms of grinning and bearing them, but in terms of creativity, then the meaning of the situation and the decision has to be discovered. Helen Oppenheimer (1995) argues that 'mattering is more given than chosen' (p. 60). Most of the issues in life that challenge us are things over which we have little control, such as accidents or events that confront us. Therefore, how we adjust to these is not only an ethical challenge but also a psychological, spiritual and emotional challenge. The question of what meaning there is in a situation is thus at the heart of such a situation. This has often to be sought, so a prior question may have to be:

• Is there a potential for meaning in this situation?

A commitment to caring, for oneself and for the people who fill our lives, implies a commitment to the potential for creativity and caring in every person.

An ethic of care is therefore committed to exploring the unusual and the unexpected. The hallmark of such an ethic is that it welcomes all, and everything is potentially creative. This needs imaginative and lateral thinking, including transcendental aspects and insights that present themselves. These help to shape the meaning of life and the changes in people's lives. It is therefore important that these features are acknowledged, heard, included in discussions and acted upon appropriately.

If we have to make a personal decision, it is important to understand as clearly as possible what makes our relationship with the person of concern unique in this situation. Most relationships are not purely work orientated or involve only friends. We have interests, needs, and perhaps hidden and unspoken agendas, that play a part and that may surface unexpectedly.

• Are there aspects that may need to be aired and acknowledged before any realistic decision can be made?

If the challenge is a situation in which someone is being helped, it may be necessary to consider a *specific* relationship of any one person with the patient or client of concern. This is far from always the most obvious person. Grandchildren, lovers and neighbours may all have a special claim. It may also be a particular nurse, a doctor or other health care personnel.

- Who may be the best person to consult if that person is not immediately available?

When the many and varied aspects of the choice in a situation have been gone over carefully, an end may be in sight:

- Is a consensus emerging?
- If not, who will have to make a decision?

At this stage it may become clear that more issues are involved than were at first evident. If this is the case, and they conflict, it may be better to look at them separately and go through the various aspects again, asking specifically 'What is happening?' and listening carefully for the answers that emerge with each one. At every stage it is important to ask and answer the following questions:

- What else is there?
- Has anything not been said or discussed yet?
- What are the possible blind spots that have still not been considered?

Having studied the problem so far, it should then have become clear how to resolve it. The fitting answer should have emerged. Indeed, it may not now seem to be 'a problem' any more, but the next logical step. Very often, the journey is (or was) as important as arriving at the goal.

STEP THREE: WHAT IS THE FITTING ANSWER? (IMPLEMENTATION)

When the foregoing questions, in particular, 'What is happening?', have been asked and answered in every possible way, then the 'fitting answer' should have emerged. It is not necessarily the 'right' answer, but the one that is relevant to *these* people in *this* situation.

To decide ethically is moral ability; to act ethically is physical ability. Decisions not only have to be taken, they also have to be implemented. To put theory into practice is often the most difficult part. If it was a decision to turn off a machine, then it has to be done, but there is more to the act than simply turning a switch. It can, and should, be done in the most caring way possible. The most appropriate person should do it in the most appropriate way.

Every caring act is an ethical act. Every nurse can give an injection, but it is *how* the injection is given that counts.

Decisions may concern the workplace and strategies for caring or acting differently. It may be necessary to establish timetables or goals and strategies on how these can be achieved. Indeed:

• Is it now a question of putting into action a moral decision, or not acting immorally?

If all aspects have been considered, the 'fitting answer' is obvious and it is also obvious how the action is to be carried out.

STEP FOUR: WHAT HAS HAPPENED? (EVALUATION)

The evaluation of any action is crucial, but it is rarely easy.

If the decision was that active treatment should be stopped for a dying person, then presumably the person will die. How the death took place and how the family reacted may then be taken as an evaluation.

If it was decided to treat a severely disabled baby at birth, then an evaluation can be made only years later, when the quality of life of that person and of the parents will be evident. Between these two extremes lie a host of other situations that will have less obvious outcomes, but nonetheless important ones. The most difficult situations are always relationships. How they are upheld, mended, ended or lived with are practical outcomes of decisions that involve choices based on values and principles. One particular situation may guide a person for life in how subsequent decisions are made.

The people who have gone through the decision-making process together should ideally also be together for an evaluation session, to consider what has happened to them and their decision. This may not always be possible. Some of the questions that may also help an evaluation could be:

• Has the decision solved the problem? If not, why not?
• In what way has the solution of one particular problem affected

the wider issue?
- Were the expected outcomes realistic? If not, why not?
- Were only particular aspects realistic? Which ones were they?
- Why were some aspects not realistic? What happened?
- If you had to decide again, would you decide in the same way? If not, why not?
- Has a greater good been achieved?
- Has this been the fitting decision? If not, why not?
- Which aspect of the decision-making process has been most helpful? Least helpful? Why? What happened?
- Which ethical aspect has been most challenged? Why?
- Which ethical theory or principle has been most helpful? Why?
- Which ethical theory or principle was irrelevant? Why?
- Have any people or relationships been hurt? In what way?
- What could have been done to avoid this?
- Has the process been difficult, complicated or painful? Why?
- Have other people also benefited from the original decision?
- Have further similar decisions been easier to make because of this one?
- Has any aspect of this ethical decision now become a universal law?

The importance of evaluation of ethical problems cannot be overstated. In nursing there is a tendency to bumble from crisis to crisis without learning much from each one. When it is possible to learn from one problem, the next decision may not be easier because it is necessarily different, but the process may be less traumatic, and more inclusive and creative. Experience is a vital aspect, especially in the area of ethics where someone's ethical competence enables all who work with that person.

An ethic of care is concerned with the present, the past and the future. Only in this way can the greater or whole picture be seen and experienced. Any evaluation will have to be seen in this wider context. We learn from what has happened.

- What has been gained by this decision?
- (How) is the person now 'more' a person?
- How can this help others in similar situations?
- What has changed for the wider community of people involved? How do they now feel, or cope? What meaning is there now for them in what has happened?
- Have any earlier fears been allayed?

• What of all the feelings expressed: how have they changed, and to what?

These are only some possible questions to guide someone in the direction of ethical thinking. In most situations such questions are at best theoretical because the situation cannot be fitted to them. Those involved in decision-making processes have to approach each situation afresh. This is perhaps the real challenge of ethics.

8

Ethical dilemmas

PROBLEMS, DILEMMAS AND AN ETHIC OF CARE

The difference between a problem and a dilemma is that a problem has a potential solution. A dilemma does not; there is only a choice between two (or more) equally difficult, bad or impossible alternatives. This is the case with many of life's situations. Any possibilities offered have equally unbearable consequences. In essence, there is no choice. Many of these situations concern the beginning or end of life. This is made all the harder when it concerns the lives of people around us, and those we are responsible for or responsive to.

Some of the dilemmas around the beginning and end of life are looked at here. Only some of the best-known topics are touched on in this field of growing importance and controversy.

When considering ethical aspects in health care, most people think immediately of abortion or euthanasia. Both are concerned with the notions of how and when life starts and ends, the quality, value or sanctity of life, the meaning of life, and our right of control over life. Life is that which we all have in common; anything that touches life generally therefore also touches us. More specifically, we will always consider our own lives and prospects when we see or hear what happens to others.

An ethic of care must surely be most appropriate at times and in circumstances where either ethics or caring are most vulnerable. The importance of the relationship between care-giver and care-receiver has been stressed strongly throughout this book. In situations of actual human dilemmas, the real human dimension of relationship should therefore be considered as a vital aspect of the debate. This is never easy because it is intangible, not measurable, and has no basis in law. Against this can be said that the person who is the significant protagonist is, in the end, always left with feelings. Since a choice has to be made, there is an act done (an abortion, a ventilator unplugged) and that will mark the person concerned. The memories left are expressed as feelings, often of guilt, loss and perhaps incompleteness. They mark the person and perhaps that individual's relationships with others and indeed himself or herself. Feelings are intangible and 'irrational' in the sense that they cannot be rationalised, but they are not wrong; they simply *are*, and because of that they are important. In caring, they matter equally in the tangible and rational aspects, and need to be taken into account when considering present dilemmas and the holistic care of people who may present years later, perhaps, with a completely different health problem.

It is beyond the province of many nurses to enter into philosophical discussions about the beginning or the worth of life, especially when working under pressure. Nurses do, however, need to be aware of their own values of life and living, especially in situations where these are questioned.

Much has been written about the concept of 'person' or 'personhood', and the distinction between 'person' and 'human'. Some of this is necessary to make adequate laws, but much of it is theory and speculation, and is of little use when caring for an actual person with a real need. In such situations, Geoffrey Hunt (1999) suggests that we consider again our attitudes when we use certain expressions. He asks if there is a difference when we use the words 'unborn child' or 'embryo', 'baby' or 'fetus'. '[T]he contrast in each case is not between the moral/emotional and the scientific/rational but between one set of reactions and attitudes and another. One is not superior to the other. They have different and, within proper bounds, legitimate roles' (p. 52).

Although Hunt writes about abortion, the same concepts can be applied to end-of-life situations. Is it a 'person' or a 'patient', 'my darling John' or 'a body' that is being cared for? It may all be the same person, but the way we see and approach the human being in need matters. This is where our own understanding of ethics and morality becomes obvious to ourselves and others. One way of seeing is not better than another, and both may change; what matters is that we see and hear the nuances and respond to the persons concerned, not to the theory behind the words only.

AT THE BEGINNING OF LIFE

Abortion

Abortion must be the oldest regularly performed operation, often with drastic results. Abortion itself is no longer the moral problem it once was and the procedure is generally accepted, even by people who belong to churches who proscribe abortion on moral grounds. Despite this, it remains one of the topics always mentioned in discussions about ethics in health care.

Data from various end-of-year censuses indicate how many abortions were carried out. In England and Wales there were 185 375 legal abortions carried out in 2000, an increase of more than 2 000 on 1999. The indication is that about 17 women per 1 000 of reproductive age have had an abortion (Craig 2001). According to Kenny Craig (2001), the high numbers and the increases are due partly to women coming from countries such as Ireland where abortion is illegal. The equivalent numbers for Korea are that about 60% of married women experience induced abortion each year, mainly because of the failure to use contraception (Um 1999).

The Abortion Act, 1967, originally allowed termination of pregnancy up to the 28th week of gestation, but this was reduced in 1990 to 24 weeks. The ethos of the Act is to save life and prevent suffering. The conditions set out for this in the Act are so worded that wide interpretation is possible.

One certain reason for the increase in abortion is that women use less hormonal contraception than they used to, but lack the knowledge to use barrier methods effectively. Media myths about contraceptives can frighten people and they lose confidence in their use. The Government is also trying to reduce teenage motherhood, and abortion is more often a subject for discussion in women's magazines. With more and better information about pregnancy, contraception and abortion, and women making life-style and career choices, the increase in abortions carried out is not surprising. Despite this, the pro- and anti-abortion lobbies are very vocal. The anti-abortionists can easily express their message in sound-bites of 'abortion is killing, killing is bad, abortion is bad'. However, the pro-abortionists 'have a more complex argument to get across – not just the right of a woman to decide, but also the tangle of moral, personal and social factors involved in a decision to have an abortion' (Whyte 1997, p. 16). The main reasons for the debate are the questions of when life begins, and the worth of the life of either the mother and/or the fetus.

Anti-abortion groups base their arguments on the unquestioned principle of the sanctity of life. This makes it difficult to reason for the saving of the mother's life, or to consider the kind of life that either mother or baby will have. Sanctity, or sacredness of life are religious terms, but they are also implicit in the Hippocratic tradition. In the controversy about abortion they are often used to imply an absolute prohibition on the taking of life, or that life should be protected absolutely. Ethical principles exist to *assert* human life and to protect it, but they are not absolutes. Society, through its laws, works out the conventions and rules that make these principles operable in practice.

Pro-abortion groups are often feminist in outlook and base their assumptions on the principle of individual freedom, and on general human rights, in particular the right of the woman over her own body. They maintain this right so absolutely that they tend to argue it to the point of disregarding a growing fetus altogether.

Nurses rightly feel that abortion is an issue of ethical debate for them. They are concerned with preserving and enhancing human life, not destroying it. The 'conscience clause' (subclause 2.5) in the Nursing and Midwifery Council Code (2002) means that nurses can opt out of taking part in an actual abortion, but those working in a gynaecological ward are still duty-bound to care for a woman before and after the operation.

Nurses in gynaecological wards have most contact with patients who have abortions. The operation is quick, so patients rarely need to stay longer than a day. Abortion is possible on demand; many of the women undergoing abortion are young (even very young) and some appear regularly on the ward. This makes one question the personal and social background of these patients, and it is easy to judge and label them. The caring relationship may therefore be fleeting, which is often unsatisfactory for nurses.

To have an abortion is always a decision made under duress. An unwanted pregnancy is an enormous emotional burden. For many women the proposition presents itself without them having thought about the moral implications beforehand. Having to make a decision quickly does not allow them time to think and talk enough. The main factor is the operation itself. It is therefore not surprising that many women suffer emotionally for many years after an abortion, often silently, because they are ashamed or feel guilty, or simply because no one else knows about it and so they dare not talk about it.

At the bedside of a woman undergoing abortion nurses need, therefore, to demonstrate a special kind of insight into the pressures that may have led to the decision. Many women are well aware of their inadequate reasoning or possible mistakes, and caring for them ethically means caring for them sensitively and creatively. This may sound paradoxical in the circumstances; it may also be the beginning of a good recovery process.

It may not be at the bedside that nurses help a person to understand the implications of abortion. Nurses in family planning clinics, as tutors, and as colleagues, however, may be called upon to help someone to decide whether to have an abortion or not, or they may personally have to make such decisions for themselves. Under pressure, the thoughts are never too clear, and the issues and feelings are perhaps too entangled to make a decision that could then be reversed the next day. Nurses may meet women who, in later life and with other health problems, may need to talk about an earlier abortion; it may be then that they can help with guidance and insights to resolve issues that may have been unfinished.

Despite these facts, it is useful here to look at abortion in the light of the decision-making process (see Ch. 7) and assume that this is done to help someone to decide whether or not to have an abortion. Although a situation where abortion is a possibility often presents as a dilemma that has no satisfactory choice or outcome, any decision-making 'process' may appear to be unrealistic. The questions that are possible with such a process are nevertheless a tool for considering the various aspects and options. The model set out in Chapter 7 may therefore be the most useful tool for starting a realistic discussion, and perhaps lead to insights and a more considered decision. It will also show that the people concerned are caring and responsible.

Step one: What is happening?

- What is happening?
- What has happened to make this a dilemma?

- Who is involved? How?
- What are the main needs of each person?
- What makes this situation an ethical dilemma?
- What moral and religious values are important in this situation, and/or elsewhere in the person's life?
- Has the person had to make a very important decision before? What was it? How had she handled it then? What was the main outcome then? What can be learnt from that for now?
- Is it a question of priority of life of the mother or of the fetus?
- Is it a question of rights of either the mother or the fetus, or one over the other?
- Does the woman feel she has a relationship with the fetus? Does this influence her? How?
- What are the feelings experienced, as far as is known, by:
  —the mother
  —the fetus (if possible)
  —the father
  —the helper
  —the immediate circle of family, friends, and/or supporters?
- How do these feelings influence what is happening?
- How do the feelings help/hinder?
- If it is a question of the value or sanctity of life, what is it that makes it so? In what way?
- In terms of good and right, what counts as good, or not good, as right, or not right, as being good, or not being good, as doing right, or not doing right?
- Is there a consideration of justice here? Is it a question of money, access to a clinic or hospital, speed, or other people and resources involved?
- Is it a problem of truth telling or honesty? In what ways is this obvious or not, necessary or not?
- Is it a problem of individual freedom with regard to (a) the mother and (b) the fetus? What are the main issues?
- Which of these principles is particularly important here? Why?
- Have all the aspects been examined, or does anything else need to be said?

This stage may be made more complex because the debate about prenatal life also includes the question if it is one life or two that have to be considered. This may need to be kept in mind and addressed more specifically.

Step two: What would happen if...?

At this stage, when everything has been laid out as facts, the need is to look to the future. A dilemma exists of two equally unsatisfactory possibilities and/or outcomes. It is therefore important to see both outcomes as clearly as possible, to speculate as much as possible, and ask what may happen if any particular course were followed.

- Could there be other options?
- How may the main persons involved feel in 6 months, 1 year, 5 years? In either case (i.e. having an abortion or not)?
- Is it a question of duty (i.e. what ought to be done as a citizen, mother, daughter, nurse, etc.)? What obligations are there, and to whom?
- What will the consequences be, as far as can be ascertained or envisaged? Can people live with the decision? If not, why not?
- Who will be gaining what from which decision?
- Who may be hurt, and how?
- What is the most creative or humane response? Could it be used to help others?
- What can be done now to lessen the emotional impact later?
- Could someone else's experience help?
- If an abortion is the decision, where, when, how is it to be? What arrangements need to be made?
- If the decision is not to have an abortion, what arrangements need to be made?
- Who needs to know of the decision?
- What other aspects, so far not mentioned, could be important?
- How has the decision to be carried out, when, by whom, or where?

Step three: What is the fitting answer?

If all the earlier questions have been asked well and answered well, then the decision, or 'fitting answer', will have emerged and the person will feel satisfied. The need is then 'only' to carry out what has become obvious.

Step four: What has happened?

In this case, the evaluation will start immediately after the decision is made. The abortion itself should present no problems, but the feelings surrounding it will be left with the person. Assuming that the operation went well:

- What feeling is the person experiencing?
- Is this a normal reaction?
- Is she feeling as she thought she would? If not, what has changed?
- Is the support sufficient?
- Has it helped to work through the decision making in this way?

There may be different aspects that are not outlined here but that are important, or those mentioned here may not be relevant. What matters in any situation is that, as far as possible, the caring and the relationship is helpful, responsible and creative. This means that the person can live with the decision and will not suffer through coercion or lack of interest.

It is never possible to be categorical about any personal matter. Abortion is personal, and it is also legal. However, that does not make it ethical or right for a particular person. Perhaps the only categorical thing that can be said is that, as professionals, we should not take part in illegal abortions.

Fetal abnormalities and diseases

The statistics given above about the number of abortions carried out each year make no distinction between abortions for unwanted pregnancies and those carried out for therapeutic reasons. Research in embryology has made significant advances and genetic abnormalities in a fetus can be diagnosed early. When parents are informed of such a possibility they are given the choice of an abortion. Hereditary diseases transmitted through, or affecting, one sex only can be detected at a very early stage of an in-vitro fertilization and it is therefore possible to transfer only the non-affected pre-embryos to the mother for gestation. These practices are laudable, but like all such processes at the limits of life, they have an ethical dimension. Science is always ahead of ethics, and ethics is ahead of the law. It may therefore be a very long time before some regulations are in place for certain conditions or treatments. In the meantime, the people concerned have to make decisions for which they may be totally unprepared, or against huge pressures exerted by health-care personnel. Two examples follow.

A case study (Anonymous 1999) describes how a 41-year-old woman and her partner 'went through psychological hell' after being given distressing information and advice concerning her pregnancy. A series of events that showed how discontinuity of care, and concern for missing test results rather than the person, made the woman believe that she may be carrying a child with Down's syndrome. She was given details of how termination takes place before she and her partner were given any explanation or interpretation of the results of a scan. An ultrasound scan carried out privately revealed no abnormalities. However, the couple 'experienced unnecessary grieving and trauma that were associated with system failures' (p. 252), and assumptions were made that she would have an abortion without questioning her and her partner's concerns, values, or feelings.

Similarly, Ann-Marie Begley (2000) describes a couple who had undergone fertility treatment, with the woman finally having a positive pregnancy test. The first scan showed that she was in fact carrying seven live fetuses. The couple were recommended to undergo multifetal pregnancy reduction. Faced with such a dilemma, the woman was determined that she could not live with the possibility of killing four fetuses to give three others a chance to develop. Her husband was strongly in favour of the reduction.

Both examples show how couples are often thrown into confusion by unexpectedly having to face decisions that will affect their whole lives, yet they are given little or no help in reaching such decisions. On the contrary, health-care professionals expect them to accept their recommended actions, which may be based entirely on science and technology rather than on ethical or human values. The couple in the first example were able to discuss their concerns with their GP and in this way obtain a second opinion, but this is not an option for everybody. It is all the more important that specialist nurses should be working in areas where life-and-death decisions have to be made or where unexpected emotional upheavals are common. Such nurses need to be well educated in the use of the technology involved, and also in decision-making processes and ethics.

Some of the concerns often voiced about the newer technologies, especially in the area of fetal diagnosis and abnormality, are:

- Is there not a danger of the creation of a 'super-race' (with the Nazi experiments still in living memory)?
- Is it right to invest vast sums of money in practices that at best benefit only very few people?
- The routine abortion of fetuses found to have abnormalities may lead to even further shunning of disabled people, and of parents who allow such a child to be born.
- Genetic screening and diagnosis can lead to 'designer babies', screened for diseases and/or physical attributes. This may be in the parents' interest, but is it also in the interests of the child so created?
- Children have been created to serve as donors of blood or stem cells for sick siblings. Is this not too much of a utilitarian approach to life and medicine? (Anonymous 2001a)

Such questions and concerns may never have satisfactory answers. Economy, efficiency and effectiveness, if seen only in terms of money, will always be in opposition to compassion, competence, confidence, conscience and commitment. In the end it is not a figure at the bottom of a balance sheet that counts, but how a particular person was treated. Despite every advanced treatment and diagnostic tool available, babies are still born malformed and with diseases, needing care and love. Many such babies would not have survived long in the past, but the treatments available now also mean that whether and how to treat them has become not only a question of equipment and human and monetary resources, but ethics: should it be done?

- Have handicapped babies a right to life?

In a closely-argued article Helga Kuhse and Peter Singer (1985) write that handicapped babies do not have more of a right to life than healthy babies. They follow reasoning that suggests that 'to have a right to something, one must have an interest in it, and to have an interest in continuing to exist, one must be a "continuing self", that is, a being that has at some time had the concept of itself existing over time' (p. 17). Severely disabled newborns cannot claim that right, so their right to life cannot be based on potential either.

Is it ever acceptable to treat severely handicapped babies simply to see if they will survive? Surely not, but deciding where to draw the line and when to call a halt is extremely difficult.

Kuhse and Singer (1985) conclude that 'there is no fundamental moral reason against thinking about newborn infants in the way we now think about fetuses when we allow a woman to abort a defective fetus and to try again to have a normal child' (p. 20). Berit Brinchman (2000) considered premature infants ('The smallest infants are not fully developed and are therefore at a high risk of being left with severe handicaps' (p. 141).), concluding that decisions concerning their lives are often ambiguous and are frequently made on the vitality of the babies concerned. This adds a whole dimension to the debate about if children can make decisions concerning their lives.

Christopher Newell (2000) argues that much genetic technology and information is based on a mechanistic and reductionist view of the world. He asks: 'What does the "deliverance" of today's and tomorrow's children from genetic disease really mean?' (p. 229). He believes that, even in single-gene conditions, therapy is hardly predicted to be cost-effective when compared with other health-care interventions. Genetic testing may eventually drain public and individual resources, raising fundamental questions about equality and resource allocation. 'Who will be allowed to order genetic tests and who will pay for them?' (p. 229), asks Newell.

The case of 'Baby J' was well reported in the press in 1990. He was born at 27 weeks' gestation with a birth weight of 1.1 kg. He required ventilation, but there were times when he could breathe spontaneously and could also be looked after at home. It took several court decisions not to resuscitate him again when he next came to that point. The Master of the Rolls, on giving judgment, quoted from a Canadian document of a similar case:

There is a strident cry in America to terminate the lives of other people – deemed physically or mentally defective ... Assuredly one test of civilization is its concern with survival of the 'unfittest', a reversal of Darwin's formulation ... In this case, the court must decide what its ward would choose, if he were in a position to make a sound judgment (Anonymous 1990, p. 24).

The shock that parents experience at the birth or news of scan results of a malformed or disabled baby is often enough for them to either reject the child or not be able to make logical decisions. Occasionally, decisions will have to be made fairly rapidly if the baby is to live. Probably more often it is true to say that decisions can wait 2 or 3 days, by which time the parents may have had some time or occasion to adjust to the diagnosis or birth, and the condition of the child itself will have given some indication of how well he or she may survive. Nevertheless, a decision will have to be made.

The ethical dilemma is always whether to let live or to let die.

At birth it is impossible to decide what IQ a child with Down's syndrome may attain. A baby born with spina bifida or other congenital malformations may have a high IQ but be subjected to an existence that may seem intolerable, but is it so to him or her? Surely life is more than just the IQ. The kind of attention a disabled infant receives at birth may very well determine his or her future life. Is it not again the quality and depth of the significant relationship that matters and that may be the most important element in such a dilemma?

AT THE END OF LIFE

Just as the issues around the beginning of life become ever more ethically charged, so are the issues around the end of life. At the beginning of life it is exclusively others who make decisions over that life. At the end, it is often a heartbreaking battle concerning who has the right or the power to end a life if death is not sudden or 'natural'. Persons concerned often feel that they would like to have as much, or at least some, control over the manner of their dying. Dying is the last act of a person and it is what those left behind will most clearly remember. With the increasing use of medical technology the manner of dying is often neither easy nor possible to control.

Death is often something that, like illness, we prefer to ignore or consider should not be there. Death is seen as the culmination of illness and, in a way, the worst illness. As most illness is dealt with in hospitals, that is where death mostly happens. This means that death has become something with which most people are not familiar. What is not seen regularly becomes strange and consequently something to be feared.

Social conditions, at least in the western world, have improved drastically. When living was little more than misery and poverty, death was something desirable, because the afterlife promised 'paradise'.

Illnesses and diseases that not so long ago were 'the old man's friend', that is, acceptable as easing the passage from life into death, are now a mere few tablets away and no more than an occasional inconvenience for someone. Living longer means postponing death. The reality of it is still there, but because medicine is able to postpone it again and again, death has become an 'outrage' and something that should not happen.

These are perhaps mainly generalisations, but much of our society's behaviour leans in that direction. The accompanying issue is a spiritual one: what one does not have to face one forgets about. The loss of religious values and practices in the West means that death has lost its desirability and its mystique. However, other cultures and religions have shown that 'suicide bombers' can hold very different values and that, to them, their own death and that of those killed with them is glory. It is, however, unlikely that this kind of martyrdom will be generally welcome.

More difficult remains the question, and the practice, of when and how life ends in old age or illness. Cessation of breathing and heart beat are not clear enough indicators of death.

Brain death has long been one of the criteria for establishing death, mainly for the purpose of procuring organs for transplantation. However, it has also always been a controversial practice. Robert Truog (1997) has argued strongly that brain death is an unsatisfactory indicator because a large number of individuals still show some neurological function after tests (p. 29), and that 'most people find it counterintuitive to perceive a breathing patient as "dead"' (p. 33). Truog suggests instead that an approach should be made to the question of organ procurement via non-maleficence and consent. He suggests that this would also resolve 'the long-standing debate over fundamental inconsistencies in the concept of brain death' (p. 36). James Bernat (1998) has added to the debate by saying that brain death is an unfortunate term that may 'be responsible for some of the conceptual confusion surrounding a neurological determination of death' (p. 15) and that, indeed, the scholars who reject the concept of brain death have actually not formally defined death. Yet, whole-brain death remains the standard for determining death.

When brain death has been diagnosed, a person may be kept ventilated for some time, usually for not more than 72 hours, for the purpose of organ procurement. Some of the ethical dilemmas facing people are around issues of death care, not of health care. The same machines that help people to live have created the problem of how and when to let someone die.

The right to die

The concepts surrounding death and dying have become more intricate and diverse. It is therefore necessary to address several issues that overlap.

A right to die has become a more frequent demand. It applies in particular to terminally ill people who do not want further treatment. Alongside a right to die has also emerged a duty to die. This refers to terminally ill people who feel that they have no choice but to refuse treatment because of social factors, such as being a burden on their family or a financial cost to society.

In 1993, Leon Kass made some impassioned statements about the right to die, refuting the very idea that one could have 'a justified claim against others that they act in a fitting manner: either that they refrain from interfering or that they deliver what is justly owed' (p. 35). He blamed the whole idea on autonomy, which has now come to mean 'doing as you please' (p. 39). The right, however, has not gone away. At the time of writing, the case of Diane Pretty was in the news because of her request that her husband should not be prosecuted if he helped her to die. She was a 42-year-old woman with advanced motor neurone disease. This right was refused in the English courts and she took her case to the European Court of Human Rights, claiming several articles under the Human Rights Act, 1998. However, the European Court of Human Rights also refused her claim. Emma Wray (2001) had argued that there were strong indications for and against giving Ms Pretty her right. However, she went further and advocated that assistance to commit suicide should generally be prohibited, but that there should also be 'a limited extension to the right of a patient to commit suicide' (p. 21). Hard cases make bad laws, but experience in Canada has shown that a middle way may be possible. This would need to be considered seriously because there is no doubt that increasing numbers of patients will present in similar situations.

A study by Emiko Konishi and Anne Davis (2001) considered both western and Japanese nurses' attitudes towards a right to die and a duty to die, probing if patients' right to die is evolving into a duty to die. Both sets of nurses upheld the right to die, but many more Japanese nurses disagreed that there is a duty to die than western nurses. 'While many nurses opposed the concept of duty-to-die, it received more support than the authors had expected' (p. 23). Their study had included 72 Japanese and 71 western nurses, so this can at best be seen as a small sample, but the concept of a duty to die will certainly become more important in the future and nurses world-wide may have to consider their values on this topic. 'Rationalisation' and redistribution of limited resources in the health-care sector will cause people to fall back on their own resources and find there are none there either. The pressure may then grow, subtly and blatantly, to induce people to consider that there is a duty to die. The fear of being a burden is very real for many people and it is not easy to see how this could diminish in the future.

- Have we become like the sorcerer's apprentice, unable to put the broom back into the cupboard? Our technologies have come to have a life of their own. Is there a way out of the spiral of technological advances that lead to human poverty?

Living wills

One possibility of ensuring that our wishes are respected is to have an advance directive (living will). Brigit Dimond (2001d) writes that, in 1999, the Government decided that it would not legislate about advance statements, considering that 'all adults have the right to consent to or refuse medical treatment. Advance statements are a means for patients to exercise that right by anticipating a time when they may lose the capacity to make or communicate a decision' (p. 1327).

After the Tony Bland case, one of the judges involved, Lord Goff, stated that respect must be given to the patient's wishes

where the patient's refusal to give his consent has been expressed at an earlier date, before he became unconscious or otherwise incapable of communicating it; though in such circumstances special care may be necessary to ensure that the prior refusal of consent is still properly to be regarded as applicable in the circumstances which have subsequently occurred (Dimond 2001c, p. 1256).

This makes it clear that living wills are not legal documents and not legal requirements, but, if properly drawn up, they have the status of a legal document and must therefore be respected. The British Medical Association (1995) has a code of practice on advance statements, the Lord Chancellor's Department (1999) has issued guidelines for making decisions on behalf of mentally incapacitated adults, and the Voluntary Euthanasia Society has standard living will forms that can be purchased, as well as free information leaflets.

The problem is not usually with the actual existence of an advance directive, but that the circumstances envisaged may not match the situation as it presents itself. The most useful practice is therefore for people to draw up a living will and at the same time appoint a friend or relative to speak for them in case this may become necessary (giving durable power of attorney). Much trauma may thus be prevented, for patients, their families and friends, and also the caring team.

Do not resuscitate orders

Lorinda Schultz (1997) cites Asplund and Britton (1990), who conducted a study in Sweden about not for resuscitation (NFR) practices. In the country's 92 acute care hospitals there were 191 different symbols and 31 written code words used to indicate the NFR status of patients: 'Examples included red zeros (indicating no action), hearts with crosses through them, and "T" (indicating terminal care), and a sunset symbol' (p. 231). However, verbal orders were the most common form of communicating the NFR status of patients. It is little wonder that there is often confusion among staff about the procedure. Schultz (1997) points out that 'CPR [cardiopulmonary resuscitation] is unique in that it is the only medical intervention able to be performed by nonmedical staff that requires a medical order for it not to be performed' (p. 230). Indeed, the decision to place a do not resuscitate (DNR) order on a patient is as much an ethical decision as a medical one. There are plenty of stories of patients not having been consulted about a DNR order (Payne 2000b, see Ch. 3), or that relatives were consulted and instructions not written down. In the event, it is often nurses who find themselves criticised if they do resuscitate or if they do not (Dimond 2001e). Sue Mason (1997) argues that a 'DNR decision is crucial for the provision of good quality care, as the experience of resuscitation for both the patient and his/her family and the healthcare professionals is not a pleasant one' (p. 646). Indeed, Schultz (1997) describes coming upon a resuscitation procedure being carried out on the ward on which she was working, and not being aware that this was actually her uncle until the procedure was over and the patient declared dead.

For the public in general, cardiopulmonary resuscitation tends to be the great life saver. It is therefore ironic that it is not equally well known that the survival to discharge ratio is only approximately 1:10 (Birtwistle and Nielsen 1998) and that suffering and dying is often prolonged when the procedure is carried out.

Mike Hayward (1999) suggests that many elderly patients might choose not to be resuscitated if they were consulted. This was found when Eun-Shim Nahm and Barbara Resnick (2001) interviewed 191 elderly people living in a continuing care retirement community in the USA. It is often argued that people could not cope with being asked if they would like to be resuscitated or not; however, in the USA it is one of the obligatory questions asked when anyone is admitted to any health-care facility. Surely people on either side of the Atlantic are not so very different? Patients make decisions about their care, and this is part of their care.

Resuscitation is often hailed as one of the breakthroughs in medical care that is now universally accepted. If it is to be so accepted, then it can be done only with the person's consent and cooperation beforehand when the person is receiving health care. This demands discussion and sharing of information; it demands sensitivity and listening; it demands the creation of a relationship; it also demands respect between staff and patients, and between staff. In this sense it is one of the breakthroughs in care, because it calls for the kind of communication that should exist at every level of care.

Euthanasia

In the past, several terms were used for different aspects of euthanasia. While the word itself means a 'good death', the way we use it means the intentional killing of someone. Thus, generally speaking, only the terms 'voluntary' and 'involuntary' euthanasia are now used. Indeed, in the Netherlands, the word euthanasia is used only for deliberate acts of killing; voluntary euthanasia is referred to as 'termination of life on request'.

The Royal Colleges of Physicians and General Practitioners' Working Group on Euthanasia have defined euthanasia as 'the active, intentional, ending of the life of a competent patient, by a doctor, at that patient's request' (Anonymous 2001b, p. 5).

The Dutch Bill to decriminalise voluntary euthanasia and doctor-assisted suicide became law in April 2001. The criteria for voluntary euthanasia and doctor-assisted suicide are as follows:

The doctor must be convinced that the patient:

A has made a voluntary and well-considered request to die

B is facing interminable and unendurable suffering.

Criteria A and B imply a long standing doctor–patient relationship, which, in effect, restricts voluntary euthanasia or doctor-assisted suicide to residents of the Netherlands.

The doctor must also:

C inform the patient about his or her situation and prospects

D together with the patient, be convinced that there is no other reasonable solution

E consult at least one other independent doctor

F give a written assessment of the due care requirements covered by criteria A–D

G help the patient to die with due medical care

H report to the relevant regional committee (made up of at least three members, including a legal expert, a doctor and an expert in ethics or philosophy).

As before, all cases must still be reported and must still go to a review committee, but the significant difference now is that if the review committee is satisfied, that is the end of the matter (Sanders 2001, p. 2).

Included in the Bill is the provision that children as young as 12 years can ask for euthanasia. Helen Scott (1999) is outraged at that idea, but Robert Weir and Charles Peters (1997) have argued that adolescents have the capacity to make decisions and ought to be given the opportunity to participate, even in the toughest of health treatment decisions such as advance directives. Even very young children are regularly consulted on treatment decisions; it must surely be better to involve children in their care than not to do so. As always, it needs sensitive care and understanding, especially in the language used.

Euthanasia is not legal in the UK; the same situation as in the Netherlands does not apply here. In the UK, palliative care is well established and used, whereas in the Netherlands it is not. The Dutch criteria make it quite clear that there must have been a long-standing doctor–patient relationship; therefore talk of 'death tourism' is exaggerated, although abuse of the system can never be ruled out. In various ways, nurses in the UK have indicated that euthanasia is not something that they welcome (Anonymous 2000a, Barr 1997, Castledine 2001a, London Palliative Care Centre Team 2001). Other nurses (Sheldon 2001, Wilks 1999) have argued that communication is the main point in any care, and that nurses need to be involved in decision making, especially around the care given at the end of life.

Most people would agree that to die with dignity is preferable to lingering and suffering. There is not only a fine line between euthanasia and pain control, there is often also a professional line. Many nurses are now better trained in pain control and palliative care and can, therefore, accept that large doses of narcotics given correctly are not euthanasia, but are in fact good patient care.

The care that patients receive at the end of their lives is perhaps the most contentious of the ethical problems that nurses meet regularly. Nurses often feel that patients are not cared for appropriately, or that doctors prescribe tests and treatments that they consider to be inappropriate, and that they need to challenge this. Professional rivalries often come to light most obviously at this time, when patients are at their most vulnerable and doctors and nurses differ most in their respective values of care. Nowhere is the need for effective communication and cooperation more necessary than at the bedside of patients who are dying, be this naturally or voluntarily.

The term 'aid-in-dying' is occasionally used to cover all aspects of dying. It is particularly used in German-speaking countries. Many euphemisms are used for this time in a person's life, so this is perhaps one term to avoid because it is so generic and can indicate anything from hospice care to involuntary euthanasia.

Assisted suicide

The term 'assisted suicide' is generally used when a doctor supplies a patient with the necessary medication to end life as and when desired. The patient has the choice whether to use the medication or not. The doctor does not actually give the medication. Nicholas Dixon (1998) believes that there is no moral difference between euthanasia and physician-assisted suicide. He states that the 'only reason for preferring one to the other [physician-assisted suicide to active euthanasia] is the purely pragmatic consideration that the willingness to commit suicide gives compelling evidence of the patient's desire to die' (p. 29). He argues that, if killing is absolutely wrong, then so is helping to kill someone. He compares this with a situation when someone is shot and killed because of a mugging. All the muggers are charged with killing, not only the one who pulled the trigger.

Arlene Klotzko (1999) agrees that there is no moral difference between euthanasia and assisted suicide, but that 'the legal differences between the practices are profound. In the US, roughly half the states have laws banning assisted suicide. Only Oregon has legalised the practice under guidelines. There are no specific statutes outlawing euthanasia. It is simply a form of murder, and consent can never provide a defence' (pp. 42–43). All the same, Jack Kevorkian, who is known as 'Doctor Death' in the USA because of the many people he has helped to die with his 'suicide machine', has never yet been convicted of murder.

The argument of a 'slippery slope' is often used in discussion surrounding euthanasia. The opportunity is certainly there for abuse, especially when fear of death and becoming a burden are considered. Euthanasia and assisted suicide may be one of those touchstones on which we decide how we want our health services to be in the future.

Withholding and withdrawing treatment

Patients in persistent vegetative state (PVS) and the associated burden on their families raise disturbing questions for doctors and nurses on what would really be best for them, considering the usually poor prognosis (Crispi and Crisci 2000, p. 533).

In its guidance for decision making, the British Medical Association (1999) states that '[f]ew issues in medicine are more complex and difficult than those addressed by patients, their relatives and their doctors concerning the decision to withhold or withdraw life-prolonging treatment' (p. xvii). This guidance had become necessary because of the Tony Bland case. In similar circumstances, doctors should be able to consult with colleagues and senior clinicians outside the treatment team in difficult situations, rather than having to seek court approval before withdrawing artificial nutrition. Although it is easier to withhold treatment in the first instance, the British Medical Association believes that there are no morally relevant differences between withholding and withdrawing treatment.

The main contention remains whether nourishing foods and fluids count as 'medical treatment'. Many people would see foods as treatment, but not fluids.

The British Medical Association guidance does not have the approval of Parliament, but there is no plan to legislate on the complex ethical issues involved (Payne 2000b). The guidance is supported by the Royal College of Nursing, which was represented in the discussion and during the preparation of the guidance. The full involvement of nurses, patients and their families in any decisions to withdraw treatment is strongly advocated.

For every story one hears about someone finally having life-prolonging treatment stopped to the great relief of relatives and staff, one hears another in which someone became conscious or could communicate a will to live. There is no possibility of applying guidelines to all situations equally. The important element is always to hear what is involved in each case.

The two doctors quoted above, Crispi and Crisci, urge their colleagues, and nurses in particular, to disseminate good, correct and serious information about PVS and similar situations, and to help the public to understand the issues involved and the need for advance directives and DNR orders. This would represent a step towards an approach to the dilemma of withdrawing and withholding treatment that would help everyone involved to choose what is best for patients and families in such situations.

Futility

In too many instances a situation arises where either a doctor pursues every possible treatment and test, even though a patient is clearly not benefiting, or the family ask that 'everything possible be done'. Usually, the parties disagree. The patient, to whom all this happens, tends to be in the middle, perhaps trying to please one side or the other, or more likely too ill to make any decisions personally. The 'futility debate' turns on the intractable conflict between deeply held beliefs and values about life.

Increasingly, however, doctors are calling a halt to interventions that do not serve health or well-being (Morreim 1994). Patients, too, would rather live with dignity, even if it is for a shorter time, than die without hair, racked by vomiting and cachexia, and away from family and friends (M Wilson, personal communication 1998).

When doctors call a halt, it can too easily be seen as giving up on a person or because of a lack of resources (mostly money) in a particular trust or institution. When patients ask that treatments or interventions should be stopped, it can be seen as an escape, and perhaps as pressure from others not to be a burden on them. Either way, there is a real danger that wrong or dangerous motives are at play and are being exploited. When it is a question of someone having been in PVS for a long time, it is also a question of the destruction of family and social life for the immediate carers. The principle of the value of life (Thiroux 1995; see Ch. 4) is questioned at every level and in every direction.

The term 'futility' refers to medical treatment that is unlikely to achieve both a qualitative and quantitative threshold that is considered minimal. This applies to the patient, but Leila Shotton (2000) argues that '"futile" nursing care of dying patients may be both incompetent and inappropriate care and, as such, may be harmful, because it is not based on the best possible knowledge and skills that nurses should possess' (p. 140). As such, futile treatment or care 'also diminishes the value of life and inhibits the professional and personal growth of health professionals' (p. 140). Shotton therefore argues that nurses must ensure that there is good communication among all carers and between staff and patients and their families. This is also advocated by Boyd (1997) as preferable to simply 'invoking futility as a *fiat*' (p. 102). Shotton's argument, however, points to the core of an ethic of care: both parties are involved and stand or fall by the care given.

The terms 'ordinary' and 'extraordinary' have also been used in discussion about the morality of prolonging life. Extraordinary means thus take on the meaning of futility, and, for the sake of clarity, 'some ethicists prefer other terms, eg "proportionate" and "disproportionate"' (Hoose 1997, p. 93).

Letting someone die

This term has often been used to indicate good medical and nursing practice. As the above shows, this is not so simple any longer.

To counter euthanasia, assisted suicide and futility, good palliative care of patients is crucial. It has been argued that ensuring 'quality of life' is meaningless because that is every person's need in health care to begin with. Daniel Callahan (1993) has argued that 'We should begin backwards. Death should be seen as the necessary and inevitable end point of medical care' (p. 33). This is similar to Thiroux's (1995) dictum that human beings should revere life and accept death. It also corresponds to Philip Russell and Ruth Sander's (1998) 'concept of a healthy death'. They state that, since 'we have a life until the moment of death, and that health is for all, a definition of health that takes into account the needs of the dying must be sought' (p. 257). They are simply one more set of authors who write of the need to advocate for patients and their families to maintain control over patients' lives and not relinquish control to the professionals.

Many aspects of the care given at the end of life present as dilemmas: whichever way one turns, and whatever one does, it is wrong, or at least not good. Again and again the main stumbling block is communication, or the lack of it. It may therefore be useful to consider the decision making process again and concentrate specifically on the ethical and moral issues in order to highlight that situations that appear to be dilemmas may not be so, and, when there appears to be helplessness and professional inadequacy, the need for nurses to be partners in decision making is not only possible, but vital.

Step one: What is happening?

- What is happening here?
- What are the main issues that make this situation difficult?
- What appear to be the main needs of the various people involved: the patient, each member of the family or friends, each doctor, each nurse, every other member of the caring team?
- Are there obvious conflicting needs or values? What are they? Why do they conflict?

- Is this a problem that can potentially be solved, or a dilemma that does have only equally bad options? Could the dilemma become a problem with a possible solution? What stops the one and prevents the other?
- What are the ethical principles involved (see Ch. 4)? What are the moral problems here? Can the situation be described in terms of ethics? If not, why not?
- In any situation where communication is questioned, issues of honesty and truth telling are evident. Is this the case here? What are the specific problems?
- The principle of the value of life is necessarily questioned. 'Whose life is it anyway?' Which aspects of the value of life are infringed? Why?
- Is there a history to any of these needs or conflicts? What is it? On what is it based? This may take a good deal of attention, self-awareness and sharing to understand. Is there professional rivalry or mistrust within the team?
- What are the underlying values, such as family and religious or spiritual values or traditions? Are they being suppressed or questioned?
- Are there pressures from hospital or trust to fulfil certain criteria of care that may be difficult to maintain here?
- Are there possibilities for sharing among the team and/or with the significant people concerned? If not, why not? What may be needed first?

Step two: What would happen if...?

It is at this point that much speculation and trying out of possibilities can be considered. It may therefore be useful to envisage something, even if it is seemingly unrealistic. Only those who dream of a better future will believe in a better future. What would happen if...? is very important at this stage because it enables responsible speculation, considering many of the ethical and moral implications.

- What are the realistic possibilities at this moment and with the given circumstances?
- What do you want? What do you really want? What would make everything different?
- What would you need to make this possible?

- There may be possibilities of calling meetings, case discussions or ethics rounds, or requests for study groups, attending workshops and courses to learn more about any part of care at the end of life. How would these help or change the present situation?
- Sometimes it is a question of one individual being difficult. It is not possible to change others, but we can change ourselves. What changes may be possible? What outcomes may this possibly have?
- In any of these situations ask, What would happen if…? and give as realistic an answer as possible.
- It should then be possible to have a number of options and strategies available. What is the fitting answer? The answer will have emerged in the process, and the choice may be for the best or the most realistic option. It is important that any strategy is workable and achievable. What does it need to carry it out? At the end of this process the main protagonists need to be in a better place than at the beginning.

Step three: What is the fitting answer?

- The answer has emerged. Now the how, what, where, when, and by whom have become clear for the situation. The only decision left is how to implement it clearly.

Step four: What has happened?

This process is essentially a short-term intervention, but it may also be an ongoing process, with several substages or steps. The outcomes may therefore depend on the stage reached or the steps taken. It is important that outcomes are always recognised and acknowledged, otherwise the process is not valid. In Niebuhr's (1963) terms, there should now be social solidarity (see Ch. 4). This is the hope, but it may take some time to get there.

The social solidarity envisaged here is that nurses can and do contribute to any decision making concerning end-of-life care. Matthew Akid (2001a) found nurses more or less evenly divided between those who consider they are involved sufficiently and those who feel they are not. A process of taking stock of their position and envisaging possible changes, giving nurses confidence in their judgement and work, will enable them also to feel and be more worthwhile partners in care. End-of-life care is one of the most taxing work situations, therefore, if the work done is satisfactory all round, it is also good work.

SOME FURTHER CONSIDERATIONS

It sometimes seems that we live too long and therefore our dying is also too long. The subject of euthanasia is an emotive one because words like killing and murder are used for actions that describe only one side of a much wider problem.

The care of elderly people often still leaves much to be desired. Those who are also mentally ill can be particularly difficult to care for. Old, demented, but alive and often very much 'kicking', they are a burden on families and society, and often to themselves. Even when they can still care for themselves, they may have lost their friends, their interests are different from those around them, and they are dependent on those who are good enough to spare them an hour or two. They have to ask and then be grateful for the smallest service. Is it not understandable that many of them wish they could die?

Perhaps it is also that a person's spiritual or transcendent needs and values are being forgotten in this age of technology, and a whole aspect of life and death is overlooked by blindness caused by the shiny stainless steel of life-saving equipment. This may be an aspect of the debate about euthanasia that has been missing for too long. The relationships a person has with the self, with others, and with God, have, on the whole, not been used as equal criteria. In an ethic of care they are, however, at the centre. The emphasis to be considered is the relationship between patients or clients and the significant others or other in their life.

It may be possible—and in many instances it is—that just as life could be said to begin when there is a relationship between mother and fetus, so life ends when relationships between patients and their significant others have ceased. When someone has been unconscious for a long time, there comes a point when a spouse, friend, or whoever is closest, detaches emotionally from that person. There is no means of reciprocating their relationship. There is no way in which the patient can any longer 'receive'. The two cannot respond to each other any more. There is no longer a meaningful relationship. The essence of personhood is responsibility; without that, the person is no longer a person.

Someone who asks for active euthanasia for a once-loved person has a heavy responsibility. This is why such a decision is surely never taken lightly. Seeing someone suffer is immensely difficult. Seeing people deteriorate, lose dignity and literally be a shadow of their former self is also degrading to the one who watches this with increasing suffering.

On the other hand, the person who asks for euthanasia, or for cessation of treatment, may not so much be asking for less treatment as for more: more attention, more help with facing death or with living meaningfully. The request for euthanasia, both for oneself and for another, must always be considered also as a cry for help.

By saying that the relationship should be one of the criteria for or against euthanasia, it is clear that someone needs to have insight into that relationship. Someone (perhaps a nurse) needs to be so close to a patient and his or her significant person that she or he can discern what that relationship is. That person, that nurse, is one who listens, who hears, responds, advocates, respects, trusts and, above all, cares. It may be a question of doing what is right and dutiful, or would be in the best interest of all, but above all it is a question of doing what is creative and healing in this situation, between the people involved; then dying and euthanasia become 'human'. Ludovic Kennedy (1990) complained that 'the real enemy is not death — it is inhumanity' (p. 9). Surely that is why we need to start with death to understand life.

The important task is always to understand as accurately as possible the situations in which we find ourselves. Ethics is not only about the big social questions such as abortion and euthanasia, but crucially about the situation at hand, the everyday events that meet us where we are. This is indeed what Niebuhr sees as the outcome when the question, 'What is happening?' is answered correctly, responsibly and therefore morally.

9

Ethical issues in nursing

THE ETHICAL ISSUES

Ethics is now generally in people's perception. It is arguable that we have to learn it (again) only because our understanding of ethics had declined or we are no longer certain what is ethical. Alternatively, one can say that our language and ideas change constantly and we now express differently and more specifically what we always knew and did, and that more aspects of our life and living call for ethical scrutiny. There are few aspects of nursing where ethics is not now invoked, debated or applied, and rightly so.

This chapter deals with many issues arising in nursing that may at first glance appear to have nothing to do with ethics. Against this it needs to be said that all our social actions are ethical actions; whatever we do has to be considered in terms of ethics because it is done with, for and to others. How this is done defines us as either ethical or unethical beings, as 'good' or 'bad', and our actions as 'right' or 'wrong'. Some issues may be mainly practical, managerial or professional, but they all have an ethical component. To consider the following issues under the heading of ethics is therefore not only reasonable but also called for, to ensure that the ethical aspects of these issues are understood.

PROFESSIONAL ISSUES

Clinical governance

The term 'clinical governance' is used as an umbrella for a range of initiatives and measures by the Department of Health, through which the NHS organisations are made accountable for the quality of services they provide. Alyson Charnock (2001) lists these as:

'Clinical audit and standard-setting
Clinical effectiveness, incorporating evidence-based practice
Clinical risk-management and, as a logical follow-on, lessons learned from complaints
Continuing professional development (lifelong learning)
Professional self regulation
Service accreditation
Research and development' (p. 34).

The idea is to develop local accountability. In the words of the Department of Health (1998), 'doing the right things, at the right time, for the right people, and doing them right – first time' (p. 6). Clinical governance therefore governs all aspects of health care and, in many ways, nursing in particular. It is in the care delivered that it is obvious how the whole process of local accountability is visible.

Neil Snee (1999) believes that clinical governance 'could create an environment where clinical excellence is as important as financial efficiency' (p. 35). It is specifically designed to improve the quality of life and health of patients. The immediate problem, therefore is how to define what this actually means for the health-care professionals who deliver the care (McSherry and Haddock 1999) and why the Commission for Health Improvement and the National Institute for Clinical Excellence (NICE) exist. Betty Raymond (2001) has argued that change and culture are the two main hindrances to clinical governance making a difference to patient care. Everyone needs to believe that the change is worth it, that the anxiety inherent in change is being addressed, and that the extra costs generated need to be met. Raymond is sceptical, mentioning a number of ingrained problems, such as the blame culture, nurses needing to study but not given incentives to do so, and the real problems of care not being addressed at root. On this last topic, she cites the loneliness of an elderly person 'who does not want the ulcer to heal because the nurse will stop visiting'. Until primary care is delivered in teams rather than hierarchies, and until 'all health care professionals, patients and politicians learn to listen to each other, clinical governance is likely to be an uphill struggle' (p. 15).

Any change is a struggle because it needs a change of attitude. The ethical issues are about the values held, and why they are held, by the people concerned. The NHS has been subject to constant changes, sometimes, it seems, for the sake of change itself. Clinical governance is intended to be about local responsibility, and this may need to be the driving force. George Castledine (2000) argues that:

> Nurses are rarely perceived as risk takers or leaders within hospitals or other medically dominated situations. Instead, institutional policies seem insistent on keeping nurses as managed resources and in multidisciplinary teams where they are unable to assert their authority and lead their medical colleagues towards true interprofessional involvement and shared decision making. Nurses ... must now start to question the future direction of nursing and seek to maintain an understanding of how nursing's core values can be more clearly articulated and promoted in a healthcare world that has always over emphasized the medical model (p. 670).

In similar mode, Petra Kopp (2001) cites Yvonne Moores, the former Chief Nursing Officer for England, as saying that clinical governance is full of opportunities for the nursing, midwifery and health visiting professions.

- Will the professions take the opportunities presented to them? The answer may not be easy, and it may turn into an ethical answer that may not be evident for many years to come.
- Is it right to expect so much of what is, after all, an idea and a wish?

Research

Clinical governance needs research to a large degree. Research needs to be carried out, accessed, implemented, monitored, supervised and disseminated (McSherry and Haddock 1999). Nurses need to access research for the best possible care to be given. They therefore have to understand how research is done, what it is, and how to interpret it. Their own research (particularly as students) therefore needs to be of a quality that is also of use and does not only state or repeat the obvious.

Much nursing research needs to be qualitative. It tended to be difficult at first for nurses to get their qualitative research cleared at the research committee stage because physicians (as members of research ethics committees) 'did not see the sense of research protocols submitted by nurses, claiming that what was attempted to be researched was obvious already' (Tschudin 2001, p. 144). Without such research, however, would anyone believe that elderly patients really did not want their ulcers to heal (Raymond 2001), or that cancer patients can cope with their disease but do not know how to cope with the fear of it recurring? They may be 'cured' by medicine, but medicine may not be willing to deal with the Pandora's box that has been opened. In the journal, *Nursing Ethics*, all authors of research articles are asked to supply an 'application' section, stating how their research may be applied in practice or education. This not only makes the research described relevant to the topic studied but also helps readers in their own research.

For research to be useful the results have to be available and disseminated. Research ethics committees are now more aware of the support they may need to give to researchers who uncover damaging or potentially harmful practices. In such instances it should not be the researcher's own responsibility if and how the findings should be published or not. At present there often 'seems to be a large gap in accountability between the ethical starting point and the finishing point of research protocols' (Tschudin 2001, p. 149). It may also be necessary for trusts and health employers to encourage nurses in particular to carry out research that is indicated for their practice and then commit themselves to implementing changes as they become obvious.

Research itself has ethical connotations, and all nurses need to be aware of these. The Declaration of Helsinki, updated in 2000 (World Medical Association 2000), is binding on all whose research involves human participants. This includes nursing research. A copy of the Declaration should ideally be given to students, together with the Nursing and Midwifery Council (NMC) *Code of Professional Conduct* (2002).

All research with human participants has to ensure that they are not harmed. There have been famous cases where harm has been caused (MacInnes 1999, Noble-Adams 1999), and the situation at Alder Hey Children's Hospital in Liverpool, where children's organs were removed at post mortem without their parents' consent, has cast a long shadow over research in the UK.

Research with children should be undertaken only if it will directly benefit the children concerned (Dimond 1999a).

The vitally important element is that research participants must give their consent voluntarily. Without such an assurance the research is clearly invalid. This demands an autonomous reasoning capacity on the part of participants, who therefore need to be selected carefully. They must also be aware that they can withdraw from the research at any time without infringement of any rights. Written consent is now the usually agreed norm, but it is not absolutely necessary in every case. The signature is not the criterion on which any judgement would be given, but rather the person's understanding of the issues involved (see below).

The information given to participants has to be clear, honest and without bias, and must be understood by them. Confidentiality (see below) and privacy must be assured and adhered to. Participants must also be assured that the research results will be made public, even if not published, depending on the circumstances. Many people are willing to be part of research even if it is difficult for them, in the belief that it will help someone. This 'gift' must be respected and honoured.

All research has to be cleared by a local research ethics committee or a multicentre research ethics committee. Most centres now have clear guidelines on how the proposals have to be presented and the protocols that have to be followed. Before any research is undertaken, researchers should ensure that they are not simply repeating earlier work, and that their work can indeed contribute to knowledge and practice. Any local guidelines and policies must be adhered to. Most nursing associations (e.g. Royal College of Nursing (RCN)) also have guidelines to help researchers, and any supporting publications or policies should be consulted.

Writing good research articles is not easy. Journals are full of articles that indicate years of work and study, but are dull and uninspiring in the way they have been written. If research is exciting, this should be conveyed in the way the results are presented. With the wide dissemination of literature, even the humblest article may be read and used in remote parts of the world. The responsibility for writing clearly, attractively and enthusiastically rests as much with educators and tutors as with students. Encouraging colleagues and students to disseminate their work and ideas is perhaps one of the best ways of ensuring that good practice is made evident.

- Research is vital for any practice, especially in health care. Equally vital is that the process of research is carried out ethically in every aspect. This demands above all that the researcher is a person of integrity who respects the people with whom the research is done and promotes their dignity.

Evidence-based practice

All practice has to be based on some evidence. Evidence can be based on research, experience or theory that is not research based, gathered from clients or patients and/or their carers, role models or experts, or passed on through policy directives (le May 1999). Vast amounts of information are easily accessible via the Internet and specific databases. Once the information is available, it is important to know how to understand, interpret and appraise what is written and read. This is a process that has to be learned and practised. Evidence-based practice is a tool for change, with clinical effectiveness as its projected outcome. Practitioners who do only as they are told, or were once taught, cannot be said to be professionals; the hallmark of professionals is that they are able to make professional decisions and be accountable for them. This in itself is evidence-based practice.

Guidelines for care

If clinical governance is to work properly, it has to include evidence-based practice. It is therefore not surprising that moves are under way to measure care outcomes. In November 2001 the Audit Commission published a report entitled *Acute Hospital Portfolio: Ward Staffing* (Audit Commission 2001). The report is critical of how trusts vary in the amount of money they spend on staffing; some spend considerably more than others. However, according to Mulholland (2001) those trusts that spend more 'tend to employ more staff per bed rather than fewer and more expensive staff. These trusts need to establish whether higher numbers of staff mean a better service for patients' (p. 11). Linking input to outcome 'would help to demonstrate value for money and determine appropriate staffing levels'.

Is such a proposal realistic? How much does it cost to give a bedpan and does it depend on what is taken away in the bedpan? How much does it cost to wipe a tear away? Nurses have always argued that it is professionally and ethically difficult to decide if one patient should get much care or several patients get some care when staffing is low. There is (too) much recording already, and this kind of measuring would certainly require more. It is questionable if everything should always be seen in terms of 'value for money'.

NICE has also called for guidelines eventually to cover all care. The RCN Institute in Oxford is a NICE-backed centre for nursing and supportive care, and has to date developed guidelines for the prevention of pressure ulcers, the assessment and prevention of falls in elderly people, and the management of violence in psychiatric inpatient units (Akid 2001b).

The issues considered so far are not only facts of life, but, by their existence they question our very being as professionals. It is not only a question of if we accept changes, guidelines for practice and care, etc. or not, or like them or not, but what we do with them. Do we engage with them or let them be? If governments can write documents about the future of health care without even mentioning nurses, then we should not only be concerned, but deeply disturbed. Why has nursing allowed this to happen? More urgently, what are nurses and nursing *now* doing to correct this?

- Guidelines and policies challenge the clinical work and professionalism of individual nurses. They also challenge the values of nursing as such, and that may have much wider implications, both positively and negatively. Is there something that ought to be done about it?

Professional regulation

The United Kingdom Central Council (UKCC) printed on all its more recent publications its mission statement: 'Protecting the public through professional standards'. If clinical governance is to work, self-regulation of the professions is a necessary component. Registered practitioners have to monitor themselves and their own practice. The UKCC (2001) believed that this is guided and supported by three principles: 'promoting good practice, preventing poor practice, and intervening in unacceptable practice' (p. 3). For this reason, the NMC now, and the UKCC before it, have certain duties that have normally been described as:

- Maintaining a register of qualified nurses and midwives.

- Providing a registration confirmation service that enables employers and the public to check the registration status of nurses and midwives and the various qualifications they hold.
- Maintaining professional standards and accountability, in particular through the *Code of Professional Conduct* and supporting guidelines. The NMC Code (2002) supersedes the various earlier UKCC guidelines on professional practice and incorporates them in the Code.
- Providing professional advice. The UKCC considered this to be one of the most important services it provided for any of its practitioners. Callers can be advised on any subject, or will be referred to sources that can provide information.
- Considering allegations of professional misconduct or unfitness to practice.

Professional self-regulation is therefore an important element of the government's wish to implement changes and give better care. Deborah Glover (1999) believes that many nurses are not clear about the difference between professional self-regulation and regulation: 'self-regulation is about protecting the public from inappropriate acts, not protecting the profession' (p. 30). Continuing professional development is one way in which individual nurses and midwives contribute to local and national effectiveness and responsibility (United Kingdom Central Council 1999b).

Alison Hill (2000) sees regulation occurring at three levels: the personal, the national, and the local, or corporate, levels. The personal level is the informal level of commitment and moral frameworks that guide human beings. 'At the national level the regulatory bodies provide formal explicit standards, certification, registration and wield their disciplinary procedure' (p. 745). It is the local or corporate level that interests Hill. 'There are increasing calls for dialogue with ordinary people. But this is not about increasing the numbers of "lay" members of professional bodies, it is about patients and carers having a say in the standards expected of professional practice' (p. 745). It is indeed this exchange that is increasingly demanded, not only in health, but also in education and business. The providers and the consumers are no longer two different groups of people. In nursing we have long talked about holistic care but largely not understood that this involves the wider setting and environment of care.

- Professional regulation should not mainly be about protecting the public from unsafe practitioners, but about how to promote professional responsibility, innovation and partnership in care. 'There needs to be a civic contract of critical trust, that has been reached through explicit public debate and the involvement of patients' (Hill 2000, p. 745). This public debate is part of the holistic care given to individuals.

Advanced practice

Advanced practice was officially outlined in the document *Making a Difference* (National Health Service 1999). This offered a career framework with three bands for nurses: registered practitioners, senior registered practitioners, and nurse consultants. However, there is still confusion about the titles, which is not helpful when patients meet a practitioner (David 2001). There seem to be three main titles used: nurse specialist, nurse practitioner, and nurse consultant. Besides these, ward sisters are also to some extent specialist practitioners, and their role should not be devalued by moves to register higher-level practice (Castledine 2001c).

Margie Salussolia (1997) questioned if 'advanced nursing practice [is] a post or a person' (p. 928). If this is unclear, employers may be reluctant to create such posts. In 1998, Lynne Wigens praised the UKCC for not setting 'explicit standards for advanced practice but to look at how specialist practice can embrace nurse practitioners and clinical nurse specialists' (pp. 268–269). The UKCC did not set standards for regulation before it ceased to exist, so the NMC had nothing to build on when it took over in April 2002. Helene Mulholland (2002) is not convinced that regulation is even necessary: 'Improved education and training programmes and mere standard-setting, rather than assessing, are also possible contenders' (p. 12).

There are a number of other well-known areas where nurses have made an enormous difference to care. NHS Direct, nursing development units, post-acute intermediate care units, practice nurses, walk-in centres, and nurse prescribing are some of the best-known initiatives. Many more are in place without arousing much public attention, but they are no less remarkable for their practice and success.

The ethical issues arising from this thumbnail sketch concern mainly professional boundaries: what are they and where are they? Do they in fact exist, or is each post or person his or her own assessor, guide and reviewer? What are the concerns of and with colleagues? Are any of their roles or jobs removed or blurred? What do the patients say about the role of nurse practitioners or consultants?

- Advanced practice gives individual nurses more kudos and incentive, but this should not happen at the expense of other roles or colleagues. In setting up posts and reviewing them, this ought to be considered.
- Many specialist roles are specific to diseases or conditions (diabetes, continence, asthma, respiratory medicine etc.) and it becomes easy to relate to a pathology rather than a person. Nurse consultants should lead the field in good care of people.
- Nursing development units have set examples of this and need to be considered as good role models.
- People generally demand quick access and quick answers to problems. This may lead to fragmented care and further loss of holistic care. Nurse consultants are in ideal situations to foster truly holistic care, working with people who are more than the sum of their diseased parts.
- Nurse consultants should have a teaching or mentoring role, enabling their colleagues to become experts also in their chosen field.
- Ray Rowden (1998) considered that leaders need commitment, an ability to listen to people, courage, humility, and a sense of fun. These are all ethical ways of being with others. Humility is not a concept that is high on the list of many leaders, but it is above all an ability to recognise one's own limits and to accept them. Humility can give people the ability to respect others and treat them with courtesy. Leadership is considered in more detail below.

There may also be a need for a different expert: a 'generalist nurse'. Lisbeth Hockey (2002) considers that admiring people for knowing more and more about less and less is not enough. In the UK, GPs have made a huge impact on care and have been the backbone of the NHS for its entire existence. In the same way, Hockey considers that generalist nurses have a role in the future. She may be proved right.

Mistakes

Making mistakes is the constant fear of nurses and midwives, and some have suffered grievously as a result. Betty Raymond (2001) believes that the culture of blame now evident in much of the NHS is one of the reasons that clinical governance will not work. 'Nurses are implicitly taught that making mistakes and not having all the answers is unacceptable' (p. 15). Because of the fear of retribution and dismissal, many mistakes (in particular drug errors) go unreported. This inevitably leads to mistrust. It is increasingly recognised that a witch hunt is not the most helpful way of dealing with mistakes, and that systems are more to blame than individuals. Daloni Carlisle (1996) wrote of a pharmacist who considered a different approach by saying, 'We make the assumption that people do not go out of their way to make mistakes' (p. 50). The pharmacist sent a letter of thanks to anyone who reported a drug error. More recently, systems have been put in place in which blame-free error reporting has become the norm (Kenny 2000). In his report, Kenny cites data for Glasgow Children's Hospital, where '0.15% of admissions were affected, averaging 39 incidents a year. Although only 4% of the errors were classed as serious, 9.2% required some remedial treatment' (p. 14). The main errors were made because morphine came in vials containing different strengths, and there were 16 different types of infusion devices used. In reducing the errors, nurses were considered to be part of the solution, not the problem. Mistakes are important elements for learning and for improving care, and in this way they ought to be considered positively for all concerned, though serious mistakes also need serious ways of dealing with them.

- Everyone makes mistakes. It is easier to respect professionals who admit to making mistakes than trusting them when they deny having made a mistake or simply hide the fact. Honesty remains a good policy.

Clinical supervision

As with much in nursing, an expression or a good idea can be quickly taken up and it is only later that the full impact is felt. Clinical supervision is one such idea. A profession that changes as quickly as nursing needs several different approaches to implement new ideas and push practice forward. There is also the constant problem of turning theory into practice, and how to make study and work a dynamic and engaging learning environment.

Neither the concept of clinical supervision nor its implementation are questioned here. What is more questionable is what it is meant to achieve, and how this is done. It is in these areas that ethical questions are raised.

According to John Cutliffe and Bridgit Proctor (1998), clinical supervision is considered to be fundamental to safeguarding standards of care, to developing expertise, and to delivering quality care. These authors cite many benefits for clients and clinicians. Ingela Berggren and Elisabeth Severinsson (2000) note 'an increase in job satisfaction, the development of competence, increased moral sensitivity, and a reduction in stress and burnout' (p. 124). Generally speaking, these benefits are about personal growth as much as about clinical effectiveness. It is therefore not surprising that there is some resistance to clinical supervision being introduced if some nurses see the process as a form of personal therapy in a tradition and culture where the public expression of emotion is discouraged. Anything that could also be seen as 'yet another management monitoring tool' may also be resisted (Cutliffe and Proctor 1998, p. 283).

John Cutliffe and colleagues (1998a) describe six cases of supervision and consider particularly the ethical problems encountered in them. They highlight confidentiality as the main component (1998b), but there are likely to be many more. Issues of professional and ethical accountability are described, as well as honesty, respect, valuing others, relationships that have suffered, advocacy, professional autonomy, etc. In most situations, when one ethical aspect or principle is infringed, others are also; therefore it is rare that only one element needs to be considered.

When supervision is carried out in a group, confidentiality must be the most important element. This is far from easy because group sessions are powerful learning tools and it would be difficult to disguise the identity of patients for the sake of confidentiality. Ground rules must therefore be clearly established in group supervision.

All the cases described by Cutliffe et al (1998a) have an element of 'confession' about them, describing the supervisees' sense of guilt, incompetence, shame, distress or helplessness. These situations are mentioned in terms of personal events, affecting the nurses emotionally; they therefore need sensitive handling. They also show that, in caring, it is indeed the whole person who is involved and that as one aspect—the personal—is given attention, other aspects—the ethical—also come to be understood.

A supervisor clearly needs to be a person who is competent in many areas of practice, counselling, rules and guidelines and their application, and communication. Above all, supervisors have to be role models, friends and supporters. They have to consider every situation seriously and compassionately. It will not do to dismiss someone with talk of 'everybody carries burdens of case material' or offer absolution. Clinical supervision is as much about the good elements of care and work as about the difficult, but it is the difficulties that have to be addressed sensitively and with respect.

In clinical supervision, Proctor's (1986) components are regularly used to understand the process. These have been described as:

Formative: concerned with education, development of self and skills, and reflection on practice

Restorative: concerned with support, dealing with emotions provoked by working with clients and patients

Normative: concerned with developing competent practice, the internalization of professional ethics and standards, self-management and monitoring (Cutliffe et al 1998b, p. 979).

The process of decision making described in Chapter 7 is also useful here. Four helpful questions are:

- What is happening?
- What would happen if…?
- What is the fitting answer?
- What has happened?

Accountability

Accountability within nursing, says Irene Heywood Jones (1999) 'means nurses will accept responsibility for actions they take to provide care' (p. 5).

According to the UKCC Code (1992a) a nurse is primarily

accountable to the patient and to the public. The NMC Code (2002) states that registered nurses and midwives 'have a duty of care to [their] patients and clients, who are entitled to receive safe and competent care' (subclause 1.4), and they 'are personally accountable for ensuring that [they] promote and protect the interests of patients and clients, irrespective of gender, age, race, ability, sexuality, economic status, lifestyle, culture and religious or political beliefs' (subclause 2.2).

There are various areas of accountability, such as moral (to one's self, one's integrity, or God), ethical (to one's fellow human beings, especially those with whom we live and work), professional (to patients and clients, and the profession), and legal (to patients and clients, and employers). Moral accountability cannot be demanded or measured, but professional, legal and ethical accountabilities need to be seen and understood together at every level of work (Tschudin and McGregor 2001).

Accountability stems from and rests on responsibility, but the two do not necessarily go together. Responsibility is the prior notion. An individual is able to make a decision and choose an action in a given set of circumstances. Accountability means that this action or decision can be defended professionally. Thus to be professionally accountable, there has to be both personal and professional responsibility. Not all responsibility demands accountability, but accountability 'is a defining feature of professionalism' (Heywood Jones 1999, p. 13).

The NMC Code (subclause 6.2) stipulates that nurses 'must acknowledge the limits of [their] professional competence and only undertake practice and accept responsibilities for those activities in which [they] are competent.' This is an instance where the regulatory body clearly guides practitioners in their work. The individual, however, is the judge of any particular circumstance where this might apply. It is often in the delegation of work that accountability is clearly recognised. Those who supervise students and colleagues must make clear judgements about the level of competence or skill necessary not to cause harm, and those accepting delegated work must also decide if and when they are capable of accepting responsibility. If questioned, ignorance is no defence, and neither is 'just following orders'.

Legal accountability is a field of growing importance in nursing (Dimond 2001a).

Ethical accountability refers mainly to the willingness to give care in a sensitive way, aware of the relationship that exists between the self and the client, and respecting the other person. Althea Allison and Ann Ewens (1998) describe the situation of a patient, Mrs Smith, who suffers from bladder cancer. Mrs Smith is visited by the GP and the district nurse, who both make assumptions about her need and acceptance of help, but without telling her the reasons. When a neighbour makes a further assumption about washing her laundry, Mrs Smith is mortified. She had not made a specific complaint that she suffered distress. The district nurse had not discussed the choices on offer; therefore she left herself open to challenges to her accountability (Allison and Ewens 1998).

Sometimes decisions have to be made quickly and there is no time to think the problem through calmly and logically. Some situations demand immediate action if the patient is not to suffer more. In these circumstances most nurses rely on their 'instincts' rather than on other guidelines or teaching. It is only when having to account for such action that they realise the gravity of the situation, or the possible consequences. At this point the difference between the novice and the expert become apparent. An expert will have acted with professional, legal and ethical accountability by dint of being a professional. Studentship is the time when the learning process leads to practitioners 'becoming accountable' (Morton-Cooper and Palmer 2000, p. 97). As usual, much of that learning process needs practitioners to make mistakes and to learn to ask others what they would do, although this must ensure that in turn they are not made to feel or look stupid.

- Accountability is the privilege of a professional person. In the excitement to take on new tasks, nurses may also get into difficulties if something goes wrong. Although accountability is to others, the responsibility is to oneself, and that cannot be taken away or changed.
- How can accountability best be taught?

Professional autonomy

The idea of autonomy is not often used now in conjunction with nursing, which has never been and does not aspire to be an independent profession. However, there has to be a degree of discretion, control and self-government within nursing for professional authority to exist. Andrew Jameton (1984) has written lucidly about professional autonomy, but he is one of the few who have done so.

John Wilkinson (1997) sees professional nursing autonomy as a desirable goal. In particular, 'collaborative case management and primary nursing present opportunities for nurses to put their unique skills into practice' (p. 707). However, he describes the consequences of autonomous practice as no more than 'seductive and highly desirable' (p. 707), thus not convincing the reader that they are actually practical possibilities.

Professional autonomy should be egalitarian. Patients, nurses and all health personnel are equals in their own right, and should not be dominated by any one group. Such autonomy is based on reason, mutual confidence through having listened, identification with the other, and avoidance of coercion to obtain one's own ends. In other words, autonomy is based on professional ethical standards, and this in turn is based on the relationship with the client or patient.

Rather than talking about professional autonomy as such, the wider concept of professionalism is more relevant. Professionalism means that (in this case) nurses experience themselves as empowered and articulate agents for change. 'They can have control over clinical decisions and speak up about poor care and unacceptable conditions, wherever these are detected' (Heywood Jones 1999, p. 5). Compliance and obedience are not virtues that are still praised or welcome in nursing.

Professional self-regulation is thus the way forward for many of the professions that cannot be entirely independent. This must include the ability to accommodate changes at every level of professional practice, especially the delivery of practice and education for practice. It must also accommodate the increasing consumer interests and involvement in health care that ask for greater public openness and accountability of practice. Above all, professional autonomy must mean that the profession can adapt, innovate, be relevant, lead, and challenge itself and the public by dealing with issues and cases expeditiously (Glover 1999).

- Professional autonomy is not an end in itself, but a means to better practice. Professional work is not done in isolation but always in relation to others, so professions need to work together. How we work together may be more important than asserting independence.

Patient autonomy

Autonomy is 'the capacity to make deliberated or reasoned decisions for oneself and to act on the basis of such decisions' (Gillon 1997, p. 19). The three components of autonomy are the ability 'to think for oneself, to make decisions for oneself, and to act for oneself on the basis of such autonomous thought and decision' (Gillon 1997, p. 19). The problems with the concept of autonomy (and thus informed consent, see below) arise mainly in the care of children, severely mentally ill patients, and elderly patients who may no longer be able to decide for themselves because of dementia.

Autonomy as an ethical concept is largely a western, specifically American, idea. In a culture of idealism and possibilities, a system of ethical principles that is based on the supremacy of autonomy and respect for autonomy is also respected. It is interesting, therefore, that in the more recent editions of their book, Beauchamp and Childress (2001) have toned down the supremacy of this principle. In the 1995 edition of Jacques Thiroux's book, the word does not even occur in the subject index. Perhaps autonomy was so highly prized because it was the one single element that could destroy paternalism, which was urgently needed. With the emphasis on an egalitarian ethic, the point needs to be less laboured.

Patients' autonomy needs to be respected and upheld, but, like all ethical principles, it is not an absolute. The concerns above about accountability are echoed here because it is clear that professionals need to assure that their decisions and actions always consider the individual person first, and do not sacrifice short-term autonomy for some other aim, even long-term autonomy. With the competent patient or client it is relatively easy to have a good and professional relationship. However, even then good communication is the basis for the relationship. In situations where patients cannot make independent decisions, much more is demanded of the relationship in terms of getting to know them so as to act in their best interest.

Although autonomy must be upheld, it is important to realise that decisions are always made in a context of personal and social frameworks. We live and work with our families or friends, ask them to help us to decide, weigh up possibilities in the light of different needs and preferences, and make decisions with others rather than alone.

The absolute necessity in order to be autonomous or make autonomous decisions is the right kind and amount of information at the right time. It is often at the end of life when such information is either not given or not respected, that problems therefore arise in respect of paternalistic actions. Bridgit Dimond (1999a) describes the case of a man aged 57 years, who was seriously injured in a road traffic accident, and who carried a card saying that he was a Jehovah's Witness and that no blood should be administered 'under any circumstances'. A surgeon decided otherwise. The patient survived and sued the doctor concerned. Sarah Breier-Mackie (2001) describes a patient who was dying of multiple myeloma and was deteriorating. He and his family repeatedly asked that his aggressive treatment be stopped, but to no avail. Autonomy must stand as an important basic element.

Has patient autonomy gone too far, however? Patients are increasingly well informed and able to assert their needs and wishes. Some health professionals find it very difficult to deal with patients who tell them which drug or treatment they need, or who know, or believe they know, what is best for them, and that they have the right to ask for it and expect it.

A Press Information Pack (undated) issued by the Jehovah's Witnesses includes a statement by a doctor that Jehovah's Witnesses as a group 'are among the most educated consumers the surgeon will ever encounter and are very knowledgeable, especially in the area of alternatives to transfusion'. The same documents state that Witnesses want to cooperate with the medical profession rather than antagonise it.

Ann McGauran (2001) describes the government initiative on chronic disease management. This states that people with chronic diseases are expert patients who should be encouraged to make 'agreements with health professionals about what they need to do to reduce unnecessary burdens on the health service' (p. 13). This is not a strategy for leaving patients with chronic diseases to their own devices, but rather helping them to 'adopt a more positive outlook on what it is like to have a chronic disease' (p. 13).

Expert patients pose a very different challenge to health professionals than did those who 'left it all to you, doctor'. Such challenges are opportunities to work together, enhance relationships, and create trust. Not all situations will be easy, but all situations can teach both sides how to enhance each other's lives.

- Thiroux (1995) puts his principle of individual freedom as the last of the principles, stating that freedom is possible only in the context of the other principles. Beauchamp and Childress (2001) put it as the first principle. Does it make a difference where it comes in a hierarchical order of principles?
- The 2002 NMC Code (subclause 2.5) states that registered nurses and midwives 'must report to a relevant person or authority, at the earliest possible time, any conscientious objection that may be relevant to [their] professional practice', but 'must continue to provide care to the best of [their] ability until alternative arrangements are implemented'. The question is how 'conscientious objection' is interpreted and what this may mean in practice.

Advocacy

Leah Curtin (1979) based a philosophy of nursing on the concept of advocacy. She says that an advocate is first and foremost a person who can and does enter into a relationship with another person. Advocacy is based upon our common humanity, our common needs, and our common human rights.

Advocacy, like clinical supervision, is an idea that was taken up enthusiastically in nursing before the concept was very clear or used uniformly. Nurses will invoke their duty to be advocates, but may mean very different things by this.

According to Mind, the National Association for Mental Health (2000): 'An advocate is someone who can both listen to you and speak for you in times of need' (p. 2). This is a simple and practical definition that could easily be adopted generally.

Advocates need to know a great many things about the persons on whose behalf they speak, and also about the reasons why patients or clients need to be spoken for in this way. Advocates have to have a good understanding of the 'common humanity' that largely corresponds to the 'reciprocity' of earlier chapters. They have to know the patients' or clients' needs, which means a receptivity that can come only from listening and hearing, and an empathy that goes beyond the superficial wants of either party involved. Thirdly, advocates need to know the human rights involved, which points to the 'responsivity' mentioned so often already. To know the rights and see the needs is one thing; to do something—to respond in a caring and ethical way—is quite another. There needs to be a courage that is born of compassion; otherwise all talk of advocacy is simply window-dressing.

In Curtin's (1979) view, nurses 'must – as human advocates – assist patients to find meaning or purpose in their living or in their dying' (p 7). In this perspective, advocacy is a synonym for caring. Advocacy and caring both demand listening, have a basis in the relationship, and demand compassion, competence, confidence, conscience and commitment.

Helga Kuhse (1997) argues that nurses do not have a moral voice of their own. She believes that, because doctors make the important decisions and nurses carry them out, this leaves them in a position where their moral point of view is lost; therefore, to be heard at all, they have to take on the patient's moral voice. That may have been one reason why nurses took on the idea of advocacy so wholeheartedly; finally there was a chance to have a voice that was legitimate. Advocacy in nursing may therefore be little more than professional rivalry, using the vulnerability of patients as an excuse to have a voice.

Advocacy is therefore about power. Kevin Teasdale (1998) agrees with Kuhse, but goes further by saying that advocacy is about 'influencing those who have power on behalf of those who do not' (p. 1). This means that those who do the influencing also have power because they can do the influencing or they can decide not to do so. There is a sense in which everyone in an institution needs to look after their own interests, otherwise the structure will not work. They can ensure that those who are powerless stay powerless. Power is a two-edged sword.

Advocacy can therefore be seen in terms of 'fighting the system'. If the system were good, patients would not need advocates. 'The system' ensures that there is an imbalance between those who are vulnerable because of illness, lack of knowledge or limited legal or consumer rights, and those who can easily become used to acting paternalistically because of this.

Student nurses can be in situations where they can see much more clearly than their institutionalised colleagues when a situation may need advocacy, but they may not be in a position where they can be effective as such; they are junior nurses with little or no contact with doctors or involvement in treatment decisions. They may also argue that those who exhort them to be advocates are the nurse academics who are not involved in day-to-day patient care.

A case study (Anonymous 2000b) tells of a student nurse who was invited into a patient's single room to see a new piece of equipment. A portable bath on loan from the intensive care unit was being demonstrated. 'Several nurses trooped in and out in order to view the new bath and to see how it handled.' Nobody seemed to consider the male patient who was naked in the bath. 'It was as if his body had become an unimportant object, secondary to the magical bath' (p. 63). The student nurse was acutely aware of the patient and was embarrassed for him, but was not able to say anything or do anything there and then.

Much of what is generally considered to be advocacy in nursing can thus be seen as simply giving good care.

Many nurses do not yet consider that everyday issues are also ethical issues, and that good care is also ethical care, and vice versa. If they are not aware that something is an ethical issue, how can they be advocates? What would they be advocating about?

- Can or should nurses give patients more information?
- Do patients have the right to receive from nurses the information withheld by other professionals?
- To whom are nurses responsible: the patient, the doctor or their conscience?
- How can nurses be effective advocates in situations of conflict?

Various types of advocacy are possible:

- Self-advocacy may sound like an excuse for getting involved, but perhaps the most effective way of caring ethically is empowering others. Advocacy transfers power back to patients to enable them to control their own affairs.
- Group advocacy often involves local gatherings. Speaking up is easier when with others than when alone.
- Peer advocacy is used a good deal in mental health, where people with experience of similar problems can help each other.
- Citizen advocacy is becoming popular all over the country for discussing local problems and putting forward strong recommendations about aspects of the locality, be this in health or other services.
- Legal advocacy is done by specialists representing formal settings such as courts, tribunals or complaints processes. It

may have financial implications.
- Some trusts have patient advocates who will investigate complaints or can be asked to help with disputes.

Advocacy is a widely understood term and concept. As so often in matters of ethics and health in general, it should not be assumed that everybody knows what it means or what an advocate does, but questions should be asked first:

- What is happening? This is a vital question at every level.
- What is being said and why?
- What needs to be done, why and how?
- Who needs to do what and why?

Informed consent

The idea of consent is based on the principle of respect for the person, and thus on the concept of human rights of life and liberty.

Essentially, all nursing actions are invasions of a person's privacy. Most of these actions are considered to be necessary and consent is given implicitly by going into hospital, or being treated at home. This should, however, never be taken for granted. It is not only courteous to ask if some care or treatment may be given and perhaps the time negotiated, but it is an ethical requirement if trespass to the person is not to be invoked (Dimond 1999a). Giving full explanations of what is being done and why, how, where and when, is essential and has to be offered, not given only if and when the patient or client asks.

The status of patients has changed considerably in recent years; they are now considered as active participants in decision making about their care (Sainio et al 2001). It is therefore clear that 'informed consent' does not simply mean 'saying yes', but also 'saying no'. This can still come as a shock to many health care practitioners, but should actually be seen as a compliment to them and their information giving. Kevin Teasdale (1998) recounts the case of a patient who had signed a consent form for a cystoscopy, but when the nurse came to prepare him for it, he said he did not know what the operation was and did not want it carried out. The nurse gave him a detailed explanation but the patient refused to have it done and finally went home.

Consent is more than writing a signature on a piece of paper prior to surgery or an invasive investigation, although more and more treatments and investigations are given only after written consent. Dimond (1999a) makes it clear that '[c]onsent by word of mouth or even by implication, i.e. by non-verbal behaviour, can be valid. Clearly, however if there is a dispute, written evidence is of far greater weight' (p. 31).

According to Katherine Dempski (2001) the three elements that constitute informed consent are: the patient or client needs to have all the necessary information, the consent needs to be given voluntarily, and the patient or client has to be competent. The problem is when someone is not competent (see above, 'Patient autonomy'). This must be decided in each case, if necessary with the help of the law. If a nurse knows of a situation where there is obvious discrepancy, laxity, compulsion or outright fraud, the nurse is obliged to make this known and prevent harm.

The distinction between ethical and legal consent becomes clear here. The ethical aspects of consent concern the respect and autonomy of individual persons, and that those who care for them do not harm them in any way. Legal consent rests on the competence of the patient.

Children under the age of 16 years are not able to give consent; but parents or guardians have to give it on their behalf, although the 'Gillick competent' child (Dimond 1999a, p. 39) is able to consent. Mentally ill people pose a greater problem, as do those who are temporarily or permanently rendered unconscious or otherwise unable to communicate. It may be necessary to clarify the legal status of patients or clients in specific instances. Contended situations may come to law, as for instance in *Re B* (Anonymous, 1987). B was a 17-year old girl with learning difficulties who was in the care of Sunderland Borough Council. She had begun to show sexual interest and the council had applied for an order to make her a ward of court, and for leave to have her sterilised. This was supported by her mother, who feared that she could become pregnant, and that this would be an 'unacceptable risk' for B and for herself.

- When may it be right to give patients medication or other treatments without their consent?

The right to know 'must come from a full explanation of the nature, purpose, duration, methods, means, inconveniences, hazards and possible effects' (Anonymous 1998, p. 36) of all treatments, invasive or otherwise, and of all experiments. Stories of patients not understanding what operations they have undergone, or what is the matter with them, are still common. Every nurse knows at least someone who is adamant that he or she has a tumour, not cancer, denying absolutely receiving any information that would shake this belief. One wonders what it means to have sometimes lengthy, painful or unpleasant treatments if the person does not know what it is for, and how voluntary the patient's consent then is. Using medical terms or abbreviations may be one way of avoiding embarrassment, but it also questions the notion of patients as partners in care.

The idea of informed consent stems from the Nuremberg trials in 1947, when 23 Nazi doctors were accused of crimes involving humans. As already noted, The Declaration of Helsinki is the main document that researchers have to adhere to; informed consent is the basis of that document.

Nurses are frequently involved in conducting research experiments and trials themselves, and assisting colleagues in their research by keeping records of blood pressure, taking blood samples, or monitoring patients' mental state. They must therefore ensure that consent has been given and is valid throughout the trial period. Indeed, nurses should check and assure themselves that all aspects of research in which they are involved are clear and have been approved by the relevant authority.

Research undertaken with children is particularly difficult. Kathleen Oberle (2000) and her colleagues point out that nurses working in neonatal intensive care units have special obligations. '[S]ound clinical practice demands that new treatments need to be tested but the infant research subjects are unable to provide consent … Parents, as surrogate decision makers, are expected to evaluate the relative risks and benefits and determine whether or not their infant will be permitted to take part' (p. 327–328). Nurses are in a position to support parents who decide if their child should take part in research; therefore, in any research, account must be taken of the actual topic to be studied, and the practical and psychological needs of the parents.

- After the inquiry at the Bristol Royal Infirmary into the conduct of paediatric cardiac practices there, the notion of informed consent, in particular informing parents of sick children what is proposed and expected, cannot be stressed enough.

Much of the information that patients are given in clinics and on ward rounds is not absorbed until much later. Hours or days afterwards questions may arise as patients puzzle out what the information means or what all this may indicate for their future health. It is then that they ask nurses to explain.

- To what extent can nurses add information to that already given, but which patients do not seem to have?
- Can nurses outline any options, or point to alternative treatments, that a doctor has not given?
- What burdens does this put on the patient?
- What ethical problems could this create for nurses vis-à-vis the doctor?

It is interesting to note that the root of the word consent means 'to feel together'. Consent is a legal need, but also a caring act that involves relating to one another.

Confidentiality

Codes of ethics normally have a clause regarding confidentiality. It is the essential component of any trusting relationship, especially a caring relationship. As with consent, confidentiality is both an ethical and a legal duty, and, when considering it in terms of accountability, there is also a professional component.

It is not difficult to see that confidentiality in health care often exists more in the wish than the fact. Every patient is likely to have numerous sets of health records, in GP surgeries, dental surgeries and health clinics, not to mention various hospitals where patients might have attended for perhaps only minor consultations. Moreover, any number of people in these settings potentially have access to these records. The Data Protection Act, 1998, protects all records written for a filing and retrieval system, but patient records have an uncanny habit of getting lost. Even though their content is protected by law, their loss could be potentially dangerous, in case of an emergency.

Every rule guiding confidentiality also has exclusions and, within nursing, Dimond (1999a) says, these exclusions 'are numerous, cause considerable confusion and are endangering the right to confidentiality itself' (p. 57). Sheila Gulley (1999) agrees that the current guidance on confidentiality does not address the dilemmas facing practising nurses. She blames the UKCC guidance for some of it because the '[e]xisiting guidelines reveal exceptions to the rules that are ambiguous, poorly defined, and could allow a breach of confidentiality to be justified in many circumstances' (p. 50).

The NMC Code (2002, clause 5) is clearer than earlier UKCC guidance, but it remains to be seen if this will help nurses in practical situations.

Subclause 5.1 implies that not all information given to nurses is necessarily confidential and specifies that some information needs to be shared with other professionals. This makes it clear that not every word spoken is to be kept confidential. Subclause 5.2 stipulates that 'patients' and clients' wishes regarding the sharing of information with their family and others' should be observed. It is in subclause 5.3 that the exceptions are mentioned. Disclosures may be made only when 'they can be justified in the public interest (usually where disclosure is essential to protect the patient or client or someone else from risk of significant harm) [or if] they are required by law or by order of a court.'

Dimond (1999b) has detailed what serious harm to another person means. She cites the possible spread of infectious disease and information about a psychiatric patient that was given to others. With the public concern about paedophiles and terrorists, this is potentially a vast area where information could be used and abused. The more immediate concerns of many nurses may be the carrying and using of illegal drugs or weapons. Nurses in accident and emergency departments are particularly exposed to such incidents. Health visitors and community nurses may also come into contact with many unexpected situations that may tax their judgement and actions. Local guidelines and policies should be followed where possible. However, in the pursuit of trusting relationships with clients and patients, this may often cause considerable strain and require professional quick thinking.

- How does a nurse combine confidentiality and safeguarding the lives of fellow citizens?

The NMC (2002) urges practitioners to contact the professional advice service on any issue that may have been raised by the Code and confidentiality must often fall into that category.

Professional accountability is not transferable and decisions cannot be delegated; nor can managers force nurses to give information against their will.

Article 8 of the Human Rights Act, 1998, concerns respect for private and family life. Some aspects of confidentiality are necessarily covered by this law, and patients and nurses can invoke the Act in disputed circumstances.

Nurses will hear many a tale told in the course of duty. Sometimes this may present the missing link in a person's story and may be most helpful in the care to be given. At other times, confidences are made simply because there is a special relationship between a nurse and a patient. One such case was a patient who had recently remarried after two previous divorces, but his present wife was aware only of one previous marriage. Knowing this would not have changed his care and the nurse kept the information to herself.

When in doubt, ask the patient or client. It is ethically more right to ask, and perhaps more cautious, than to make assumptions and possibly cause harm. Would the patient be agreeable to having the information disclosed? Most information given to professionals is not secret, but it is more respectful of the person to ask if what has been revealed can be passed on to the relevant authority, team, or other person, so that the patient can be cared for more effectively.

Patients have the right of access to information held in their manual health records, through the Access to Health Records Act, 1990. Access to computerised records is restricted, but under certain conditions these can be made available.

- Patient autonomy, informed consent and confidentiality go hand in hand in health care. Very often they are seen as rights that patients have and which staff need to assure. As usual, it is not simply all giving on one side and all taking on the other. Patients also have the same responsibilities. Patient contracts and civic contracts are possible only when the various aspects combine and are set within a bigger picture of a national *health* service.

Whistleblowing

Taking the advocacy role seriously may mean that whistle-blowing will follow. There is, however, some confusion between what the UKCC Code called 'report to an appropriate person and authority', and what the NMC Code calls reporting 'circumstances in the environment of care that could jeopardise standards of practice … to a senior person with sufficient authority to manage them' (subclause 8.3). A definition of whistleblowing was made by Anthony Frais (2001) as being an 'external disclosure by an individual to the public via the media. It is distinct from an internal disclosure' (p. 13). In this sense, what the NMC Code refers to is 'internal disclosure'; what nurse Graham Pink did was whistleblowing (Snell 1997). Other cases of nurses who blew the whistle have been well reported (Castledine 1997, Millar 1997, White 1998). Most nurses will also be familiar with the name of Dr Steve Bolson, the anaesthetist at the Bristol Royal Infirmary who brought to light the problems over paediatric cardiac surgery death rates (Mulholland 2001).

What may start as an internal disclosure may end up as whistleblowing if the person making the complaint is not heard or not taken seriously. It may well be that situations are first voiced during clinical supervision or mentoring. The question is then, how to proceed, or even if to proceed.

The *Nursing Times* (Anonymous 2000c) has a 'Dilemmas' column where anonymous cases are printed and experts give their verdicts. One such situation describes an occupational therapist who was 'off-hand and brusque' and 'rude' with a nurse and a patient. The nurse mentioned this to the senior nurse, who suggested that the nurse provide a written report. She was reluctant to do this because she would have to continue working with the occupational therapist. The three experts consulted in this instance all agreed that the nurse should write the report, as honestly and objectively as possible.

David Crouch (2001) asked nurses to send him stories of situations when they had taken a stand on bad practice. He concedes that 'raising concerns at work is an unavoidable necessity if nurses are to adhere to the UKCC code of conduct, it may not change the situation – in one case managers' failure to respond even led to a patient's death' (p. 24). He comments that the rigid professional structure and hierarchies make it very hard for nurses to say what they really think.

This is a sad indictment on a profession that needs a voice, wants and needs self-regulation, and is concerned with higher levels of practice and care. Nurses need to continue blowing the whistle, but they need to do this against a background (as described above about drug errors) where they are rewarded for their vigilance and respect for human rights.

- Blowing the whistle on unacceptable practice is a professional duty. Is it then not also a professional duty to follow up such acts in a supportive way?

Political action

Nurses who have made concerns known have ccme up against rigid structures and hierarchies that hinder rather than help. In their actions they were caring, and by what they found when they took these action they needed to become political. It is impossible to care in a system that restricts its workers professionally and creatively as human beings. If that is to change, then nurses need to take political action. This is not necessarily in a party political manner, but rather in the sense in which the term is used to indicate astuteness and interest in how organisations are governed and how change is brought about. In this sense nurses are involved in politics. They cannot afford not to be.

'Being political means influencing or exerting power on others, particularly in the sphere of the decision-making process' (Albarran 1995, p. 461). Many nurses feel that they pay their union dues, and therefore the union leaders and stewards are the ones to speak on their behalf. Political action is, however, often much more a local issue than a national one. It is locally that people have influence and responsibility. Because of clinical governance, the main action is at local level. Nurses need to exploit this and not let themselves be political pawns between parties and government departments.

Probably too few nurses are aware of the Green Papers, White Papers, discussion documents and reports produced by the Department of Health and various other interested bodies. Politics is about ownership of power and party politics is about ensuring that policies are defined in the interests of the dominant group. This is why many people do not like and would rather have nothing to do with politics. However, nurses who take on the patient's voice also act politically because they are concerned that people who are powerless should also have a right to be heard and respected. This can only be done 'politically'. John Albarran

(1995) uses precisely the same clause (11) of the UKCC Code that is mainly used for whistleblowing (which asks nurses to report to an appropriate person or authority any circumstances in the environment of care that could jeopardise standards of practice) to make his point: 'The UKCC implies that a nurse's duty must be to act and, when necessary, stress the shortcomings of health care policies in the institution or the community, which may also be perceived as political advocacy ... From this stance, the duty of care demands a duty to be politically responsive' (p. 463). This needs in particular the skills of negotiation, chairing meetings, and understanding how power is used as a means to influence change. It is not enough to learn this simply by 'osmosis'; it must be part of early preregistration learning and training. This may be one more topic to fit into the curriculum, and the question may be:

• can nursing afford not to be political? If it does, it may find that one day it has simply disappeared.

Strikes

The area of industrial action is difficult and sensitive. A contract between an employer and an employee implies that there are two sides to any bargain. There is a duty and a right on both sides. No nurse is happy to walk out on sick and ill people in demand for more money. Salaries are largely national issues rather than local ones; therefore industrial action tends also to be national action.

In a whole issue of *Nursing Ethics* (1997) devoted to strikes and industrial action, authors wrote again and again that they would have to think carefully about if they were to take part in such action. Most of them wrote that they would do so, depending on the reason for the strike, being aware that their working conditions have to be right for care to be carried out to the best of their ability. They also noted that they would ensure that patients would not be harmed, by manning the picket lines during their meal breaks and time off, and covering for each other's duties.

Industrial action is political action and there are various ways of making the nursing voice heard. There have not been protracted strikes by nurses in the UK for many years. Nurses in Ireland engaged in industrial strike action for 8 days in October 1999 over the structure and conditions of nursing. Jean Clarke and Catherine O'Neill (2001) write that the strike 'demonstrated the challenges that confront us in relation to caring and how we as a society value caring' (p. 357). They make a distinction between humanistic caring and technical caring; the first relating to comfort or dependency needs and the second to therapeutic needs that are quantifiable. They suggest

> *that individual nurses and nursing organizations need to work towards articulating the complexity of caring in order to educate the public and the media about the value of humanistic caring. Failure to do so may result in nurses being valued only as technical carers and in a situation where worker substitution is used as the argument for changing the practice of nursing away from humanistic caring* (p. 357).

They argue that the media concentrated on the technical care aspect of the strike to the exclusion of humanistic caring. Their statement also points to the wider value of industrial action as a political tool. Indeed, it sums up the essence of all aspects of professional issues addressed in this chapter.

- Whose ends are whose aims?
- How can they be clarified?
- Is it possible to achieve caring aims without political action?
- Some people say that caring and politics do not mix; holistic care means that a person is more than the sum of his or her parts. A politician needs care; caring goes beyond any boundaries.
- Should caring be restricted to technical skills to enable it to be measured? (see above, 'Guidelines for care').

Strikes and industrial action are always emotive terms in health care. The reasons for any breakdown in relationships between employers and employees are also emotive; therefore the relationship between humanistic and technical caring must be understood much more deeply if there is not to be a further polarisation of these parties and terms.

EDUCATIONAL ISSUES

Nurse education and ethics

Preregistration nurse education has suffered many problems in recent years. As Project 2000 became unworkable, something needed to be put into its place but it took some time until Fitness for Practice emerged and was ready. Postregistration has gone through upheavals too, as continuing professional development and Postregistration Education and Practice (PREP) began to function.

All nurse education now takes place in colleges of nursing or universities, regardless of whether this is for diploma or degree courses.

In the late 1990s the shortage of nurses was severe, and the government promised that there would be 20 000 more nurses by 2004. This meant drastically increasing the student quota. Janet Gillan (2001) believes that, in turn, this has placed heavy demands on lecturers in nurse education who 'are struggling to meet the demands placed upon [them] and worry that the quality of [their] work is being compromised.' The causes of these problems are the results of 'badly thought through policies and their subsequent implementation, and never ending change for the sake of it' (p. 31). This may be a perception as much as a fact because change is a constant necessity, and there are always cycles of expansion and contraction.

Nurses also experience problems in that employers are not generous in their commitment and support for those who want and need to pursue their PREP requirements. In times of staff shortages, this may be the first restriction placed on nurses.

In the wider context, a government that is committed to local accountability through clinical governance needs to make the NHS learner friendly. It is not possible to squeeze professionals for all their knowledge and skills without enabling them to update these and enhance their careers.

These aspects of nurse education are in themselves worrying and question the ethics of these practices.

- One practice tends to be at the expense of another. When one layer suffers, it is the layer beneath that is hurt. It is inevitably the patients who are the end-sufferers in this scenario.

It is therefore all the more important to consider how ethics is taught in both pre- and postregistration courses. It is a requirement of the curriculum, but wide variation is possible in how the requirement is fulfilled.

Ethics is a subject, but it is also a way of being a professional. Ethics can be taught, and often is, as single topics to big classes of students who have little idea of what any particular topic means in practice. Yet, ethics is about more than knowledge. Anne Tomlinson (2001) makes a telling point about students: 'Very soon after starting the course, a culture of expediency sets in. Time constraints become the dominant factor, the "need to know" takes over from the "desire to learn more about", and reading becomes directed solely towards the production of the next assignment rather than being a glorious trawl through the uncharted waters of different … approaches' (p. 3). Ethics education suffers too often from these constraints.

As ethics is about values, and 'being' as much as 'doing', the subject is ideally learned in discussion and reflection. It is in being together with colleagues that values are considered and questioned. It is in the cut and thrust of debate that the personality is formed. (Earlier in this chapter one aspect of clinical supervision was described as 'formative'; see 'Clinical supervision'.) This takes time and 'time is money'; money is what is measurable but not what necessarily makes for satisfaction.

The content of ethics education cannot be restricted to a few principles and theories, with consent and confidentiality added for good measure. Ethics concerns how society functions, the concepts of power and its use, the impact of terrorism and war on health care, discrimination of all kinds (especially ageism and sexism), the use of resources, globalisation, the use and abuse of toxic substances and the impact on society, and many more aspects. Some of these are addressed in the preregistration curriculum, but they need to be considered also from the point of view of ethics.

Ethics needs to be formally taught, but only to a certain degree. Nurses need to be conversant with the language of ethics and be familiar with some of the concepts, but they do not need to be ethicists. They need to be able to recognise when an action is unethical or when a situation may question a person's human rights. They must learn how to recognise such instances more quickly in discussions rather than by reading about them. Ethics should therefore not be taught so much as a discrete subject, but be constantly addressed throughout the course in every subject. This needs more than a teacher in ethics who gives the relevant lectures and then withdraws from the class. It means that all who teach nurses have to have a good knowledge of ethics and must be able to answer and discuss issues with students. It may mean that a specialist ethics teacher can be called upon to discuss a particular problem or situation when required, or at regular intervals. However, ethics needs to be integrated generally in every curriculum.

Every nurse is accountable for her or his practice. This accountability is at the same time professional, legal and ethical. Nurses need to understand that there is a seamless link between these three facets. If this is not taught and demonstrated practically in every situation, example or class, it is difficult to see how nurses can live it in their practice. This is another reason why ethics must be an integral part of the curriculum.

The concept that ethics is best learned in discussion has been translated into the wider field, where ethics conferences have begun to consist entirely of discussion groups, not lectures. In this way everyone can take part and learn much more than from publications that are often theoretical, technical, and leave no time for questions.

If we want ethically competent practitioners, we have to have creative teaching and learning. The content of the ethics components of curricula have been analysed (Ersoy and Göz 2001) and changed after analysis (Nolan and Markert 2002). Analyses have also been conducted to determine if nurses make better ethical and moral decisions if they are taught better (Han and Ahn 2000). This is difficult to establish because at the beginning of a course students will not have had the possibility to make decisions in the same way as they will have done after completing their clinical placements. What has been found more frequently is that, despite theoretical ethics education, in situations of emergency, nurses and doctors make decisions from 'instinct', 'gut feelings' and 'automatic pilot', rather than by ethical reasoning (Porter 2002, Rickard et al 1996). Maurice Rickard and colleagues argue that nurses and doctors use a 'two-level' philosophical view of the nature of moral thinking: one for people one is very close to (such as one's mother) and one for other people. This points to the argument that ethics based on 'feelings' is not 'really' ethics. However, these authors do not exalt one way of making decisions and denigrate another. Rather, they point to the fact that we make different judgements in different situations and need to acknowledge this. These are therefore the kind of issues that need to be discussed, especially with peers, in an atmosphere of learning rather than judging.

- If feelings override clinical judgements, can our decisions be valid ethical decisions? If yes, why? If no, why?
- Are there ways and means of getting health trusts to understand that they have a responsibility to foster continuing professional development, and therefore to help and encourage staff by giving them the time and opportunities for study?
- If nurses in the UK have problems with their education, what may nursing students in developing countries experience? Do nurses here have a responsibility to be concerned about this?

MANAGERIAL ISSUES

Senior management

Some people may argue that most ethical issues in health care (apart from those directly caused by patients' illnesses) are to some extent linked with or due to managerial structures and working. All nurses have a managerial role, from the way they organise their care of even a small number of patients or staff to being in charge of teams and departments. In considering here some issues of senior management, only some aspects are highlighted. As has so often been pointed out in this book, every situation poses its own problems and, while some issues can be understood similarly and have equivalent structures, no two outcomes are the same, not least because the people involved will be different.

One long-standing problem has been that managers did not have a code of ethics. It has been argued that management and ethics are opposing forces. A draft *Code of Conduct for NHS Managers* was issued by the government in May 2002. The NMC Code (2002, subclause 8.4), considers clearly that nurses are sometimes in management positions as it states, 'When working as a manager, you have a duty towards patients and clients, colleagues, the wider community, and the organisation in which you and your colleagues work ... your first consideration in all activities must be the interests and safety of patients and clients.' This is a very general statement and may not be helpful in the many situations in which managers find themselves that may question the way in which they work.

Valerie Buxton (1996) has pointed out that anyone who has worked in the NHS for any length of time will have seen 'the same ideas coming around again and again and, understandably, they become cynical about the whole process. Taking the wrong starting point is at the root of the problem. Patients and the public must be placed at the centre of care delivery, rather than the service being developed to fit the organisation providing the care' (p. 29). This is perhaps the crux of the matter: organisations always look after themselves and their survival, therefore their existence in terms of ethics must be questioned.

- Can organisations be ethical?

They should be, if the people who make up the organisation are ethical and consider the other people concerned rather than the institutional and hierarchical structures.

Managers, like politicians, take up their jobs because they believe that they can make an impact and can change their environment. All too soon, managers and politicians, however, tend to become part of the establishment and find that they can change little. If it were only the institutional and hierarchical structures that needed changing, that would be easy, but attitudes need to be changed, so this is a different matter.

At present, the ideas revolve around clinical governance and thus local responsibility. This means that a flat organisation is preferred over a tall one, so more responsibility is devolved downwards. Rosemary Rushmer (2000) has demystified some of the rhetoric associated with these ideas and said simply that this means that people lower down in the hierarchy are given more to do but do not receive the same salary that once went with a manager higher up. She calls this exploitation.

- Can managers challenge the situations they are presented with but over which they have no control?
- Can managers expect that their staff are willing to work with new ideas and practices when they have become cynical, having seen it all before?

There are not usually monetary incentives, so managers have few other means of enthusing their staff to make changes again. Their best means is their own example and willingness. Managers need to be people-orientated and to know how people react, work and can be engaged in practices that make sense. Managers also have to be genuine and honest because most staff have contact with them only at important moments. It matters how managers engage with staff at such times. It is in these often short interactions that it is most obvious how ethical, or otherwise, managers are themselves, and, as they represent the institution, how ethical the institution is.

Complaints

Managers will probably spend much of their time and energy dealing with complaints, large and small. The buck stops there, or at least long enough to be considered. Depending on the role of a manager, complaints may be about staff or work, the running of the institution itself, or the customers of the institution.

In the NHS a comprehensive complaints procedure is in place for patients. This was introduced after publication of the Wilson Report, *Being Heard* (Department of Health 1994). The Report recommended 'that the following principles should be incorporated into any NHS complaints procedure:

responsiveness
quality enhancement
cost effectiveness
accessibility
impartiality
simplicity
speed
confidentiality
accountability' (p. 37).

These 'principles' are also ethical aspects of resolving any conflict and they should be applied if dealing with patient or staff complaints. In any complaint or conflict there will be a large measure of hurt feelings that may have a history that is not relevant to the present situation. This means that one has to be sensitive to the present situation and the people involved, and possibly orientate them more carefully to what is happening. Feelings are often not rational, but they are powerful, and that needs to be respected. Being heard is an important aspect of bringing feelings into the present and making use of them for good.

One often hears of people saying that they understand

perfectly that mistakes are made; what they would like is honesty and an apology rather than compensation. Apologising is not easy, because it exposes weakness. Perhaps this is where managers can help; in enabling their staff to apologise when and where necessary. Saying sorry—and thank you—are small words that can make a huge difference.

- People who have been wronged or hurt often want or need redress. When this is not forthcoming, they may pursue compensation. A more ethical way may be for parties to be brought together, ensuring that people on each side are heard and can say what needs to be said. This may be costly in terms of personal effort, but it may also be cost-effective in terms of compensation saved. More is gained and learned by being human with each other (because a relationship is formed) than by money changing hands.

Leadership

Managers are leaders, and leaders are also managers. They may not always be in both roles at once. Leaders are not necessarily born; with good training they can also be 'made'. Styles of leadership vary depending on the psychological make-up of the person. Some people lead from the front, others from behind. All, however, need to have the capacity to be alongside those who are being led. Leadership in nursing is required at many different levels: in practice in wards and the community, and in education, research and management. Leaders need to be working at local, national and international levels. Clinical leadership alone is considered here, addressing some of the ethical issues that may be inherent in their role.

Alison Morton-Cooper and Anne Palmer (2000, p. 35) quote the little poem by Guillaume Apollinaire that must surely be the motto of every leadership programme:

'Come to the edge', he said.
They said, 'We are afraid'.
'Come to the edge', he said.
They came.
He pushed them...
And they flew!

Leaders have to have a good knowledge of psychology to know how they can best lead others, and what makes some people leaders and others willing or needing to be led. Alison Binnie (1998) commented that, as a ward sister, she appointed many nurses who had had a thoroughly modern education and were able to talk intelligently about the nurse–patient relationship and the impact of individualised care. However, it was not until they actually experienced patient-centred nursing that they began to 'know' what these concepts mean in practice. External and internal knowing may not happen at the same time. It is the leader's job to enable the two to come together. Jenine Willis (1999) told the story of Charlotte McArdle, who wanted to change practices on her ward. She first made a few changes, and then invited all the staff to air their views and gave them an outline of plans. She encountered the hesitation that is only to be expected: resistance, lack of confidence and fear of being asked to do too much or of being too accountable. 'Her response was to lead by example – she maintains her own caseload – and to support staff so that they could develop confidence as autonomous practitioners' (p. 34). Robert Munro (1999) told the story of Stephen Moss, who was of the opinion that leadership is 'to do with getting rid of command and control mindsets and encouraging people to be whacky in their ideas and take risks' (p. 63). Ray Rowden (1998) believes that leaders need many talents, 'including energy, commitment, resilience, the ability to listen to other people, courage, humility and a sense of fun' (p. 63). Martin Cook (2001) is convinced that there is a bright future for clinical leaders in nursing. Despite the fact that leadership has been widely researched and written about, training and development have had little impact. Cook considers that clinical leaders themselves must be able to 'focus and articulate their views, values and creativity, and to use these to improve care' (p. 45). This brings the argument back to the main point of this book; that the values that we have and hold have to be concerned with helping others to be human, that is, creative. If we are to be creative in caring, it also means expressing this in relationships by being receptive, relating, and responsive.

- How much can leaders use and express their own values in which they work?
- Do they need first of all to express the values of the

organisation they work in?

- This may lead to conflict between personal and organisational values. Which set of values has precedence?
- Can managers encourage their staff to develop in the best interests of the person concerned, or do they need staff who follow rules and cause no problems in the organisation?
- Is it enough for leaders to have commitment, courage and resilience? From where do they receive their support?
- Most ethical problems are caused by values of one kind being in conflict with different values. First asking, 'What is happening?' will provide a starting point. Then asking, 'What would happen if… ?' enables the creative and whacky ideas to develop and the possible outcomes to be envisaged in terms of ethics. Next, 'What is the fitting answer?' may present itself, and the outcomes may be seen before too long.

SOCIAL ISSUES

In this short section, three social issues are addressed that concern nurses; these are those that are the most newsworthy from among many.

Abuse

Abuse can be of various types: physical, psychological, verbal, sexual, financial and neglectful (O'Dowd 1999). Nurses can be both abusers and the abused. In particular, sexual abuse towards nurses is well known. It is also, sadly, an issue that is not taken seriously enough. Every now and again a nursing journal will publish an anonymous story of a nurse who has been abused and then found that she was made to feel that it was entirely her own fault (Anonymous 1998). The managers seemed to find it difficult to believe her story because the person whom she alleged committed the abuse was such a nice man.

The question 'What is happening?' needs to be asked in any situation, but this situation, more than any other, shows that hearing what is being said in answer is vital. Many stories may sound incredible, but if the person is not heard and believed, psychological abuse may be added to the sexual abuse.

Many people may find it easier to speak up for someone else

than for themselves. However, in nursing this seems not to be the case; nurses find all too often that they are alone and not supported when they need it most or expect it most from their colleagues.

It is not difficult to realise that nurses can be prey to sexual harassment when they have so often been portrayed as sex symbols in the press. To deal with it effectively, however, needs 'intelligent analysis and investigation and the type of understanding that could help to prevent further abuse' (Gillan 1999, p. 22).

Other well-known forms of abuse are bullying, shouting at staff, making disparaging remarks about people and the profession, and manipulating resources of many kinds. Tracy McFall (2001) lists the steps to be taken in all such instances: keeping a record of what has been said and done; telling a colleague or family member who may be counted on to be supportive; contacting the occupational health service or GP; obtaining advice from a union or professional body; requesting confidentiality until it is possible to make clear moves.

- Abusing a person in any way is often an act of insecure people who believe that they can get what they want or need by using force. Exposing harassment and abuse will never be easy for either side, but, with good handling and care, there may hopefully be a good outcome.

Racism

Racism is another topic that is never far from the headlines in nursing. The attacks in the USA in September 2001 sparked much fear and racist backlash. According to Maya Shaha (1998) three aspects are connected with racism: 'structure, ideology and process' (p. 140). Where there are ethnic divisions between groups of people, one group may want to dominate the other. Beliefs about certain groups become stereotyped (e.g. that Muslims are terrorists). Structure and ideology become reinforced in daily practice that becomes part of 'the political, social and economic system of a country' (p. 140). In western countries this can be seen in the way that refugees and asylum seekers are often treated more like criminals than as people in need. When people do not speak the language of the country they are in, or are difficult to understand, they are dismissed or become scapegoats for any number of inherent problems in society. Mary Dawood and Jo James (2001) list how nurses see refugees:

They use hospitals for primary care problems
They are demanding
Their communication/language is poor
They are aggressive
They are not employed but they are using our services
They have high expectations of the health service
There is cultural confusion
They have poor personal hygiene/clothing
They demand same-sex doctors (p. 24).

Robert Hoskins (2001) asserts that 'it's our duty to stop racism' (p. 20). He believes that nurses need to challenge patients who express racist attitudes and support ethnic minority patients who have been victims of racial abuse. Most of all, he considers that nurses have 'an ethical responsibility to support patients who have been victimised for crimes they did not commit' (p. 20).

Nurses can be both recipients and perpetrators of racist comments and attacks. Many nurses from ethnic minorities have found it difficult to rise to senior positions. One nurse was removed from the UKCC register for physically and racially abusing patients (Castledine 2001b).

- What we do not tolerate from others we should not inflict on them, or, as the 'Golden Rule' puts it: 'Do unto others as you would be done to by them.'
- Racial differences make humanity interesting, not difficult.

Complementary and alternative therapies

Complementary and alternative therapies are becoming increasingly accepted and used by many people. Some, like osteopathy, chiropractic, acupuncture and homeopathy are used by GPs and are now more frequently available on the NHS by referral. As such, they have created a popular movement alongside, and often in opposition to, orthodox medicine. This can create confusion for patients. Many nurses have privately undertaken courses, often in aromatherapy and reflexology, and are using these methods as part of their care. Other regularly used therapies are visualisation, healing, traditional Chinese medicine, and shiatsu. In addition, many food supplements and remedies connected with or enhancing certain therapies are available over the counter in shops; they are often cheap and effective.

Complementary therapies vary greatly in their application and effectiveness. Much depends on practitioners and their experience and skill. Many practitioners are not licensed or supervised, so prospective clients need to judge if they want to receive their services.

The most obvious difference between complementary therapies and orthodox medicine is the approach to the person who presents with a problem. The traditional medical model of diagnosis, prognosis and treatment does not apply. Clients may present with a clear symptom, such as a specific pain, but therapists may not be interested in the pain and talk with the person about life-style. Clients therefore feel much more heard and accepted, even if perhaps puzzled at first. There is also usually more time available for consultation, typically an hour. The often-heard difference is that these therapists treat the person not the disease, as in orthodox medicine.

With the increased popularity of complementary and alternative therapies, a groundswell has taken place that has forced those in orthodox medicine to consider holistic care and different approaches to health and illness. Many orthodox practitioners dismiss complementary therapies on the grounds that they have not been tested scientifically in double-blind or random controlled trials. Against this, complementary therapists say that their therapies or remedies work at a different level from the scientific and that it is therefore pointless to test them with a system that cannot apply. The best defence that homeopathy has is that many veterinary surgeons use it with animals, which cannot argue as humans do, but usually they improve or the condition does not progress.

- Any system that challenges an existing one has much to answer. Nurses are frequently asked about the efficacy of a therapy or remedy, especially when powerful treatments or medications cause patients to be more ill or not improve. Because these therapies are often given on a private basis, people have a personal investment and are encouraged to be partners in care and take responsibility for their own health.

This may cause a shift in attitude and nurses need to be aware of this. 'What is happening?' may again be a useful question. Listening is not only part of any care but is an important tool in understanding what a person may be experiencing, and why.

The care and treatment of many different groups of people and their needs are issues that have divers ethical connotations. Most of them are addressed in specialist texts and are more realistically considered there.

10

Ethics into the future

INTO THE FUTURE

The borderline between the acceptable and the not (yet) acceptable is always an important forum for ethical thinking and acting. What is accepted and acceptable is not greatly disputed. What is disputed is how the (as yet) unacceptable is or can be made acceptable, or not. Today, with few if any clear points of reference, ethics is shaped rather than known, and is therefore often a thing of the moment. In the 10 years between this and the last edition of this book, not only have the issues changed but also the ways of addressing them. How today's issues and topics are dealt with will shape how those of tomorrow will be viewed and handled.

GENETICS

The newer technologies of stem cell research, transplantation of embryonic material, and the whole area of cloning and genetics, have so far been echoed little in the nursing literature (Anderson 2000). This is regrettable because the voice of nursing in the debate of these issues is vital if a balance is to be maintained between technical possibilities and application in the care of people who are suffering. It is only by taking part in the wider debate that nurses can respond to the human needs encountered when the extraordinary possibilities of human ingenuity are realised.

The laudable exceptions are a number of people who have written about genetics in nursing: Gwen Anderson and her colleagues (Anderson et al 2000), who used feminist principles to argue for the need for transdisciplinary (rather than single) teams in the area of genetics; Rachel Iredale (2000), who considered the relevance of eugenics to the contemporary health care scene; Maggie Kirk (2000), who wrote about the education of nurses and midwives in the field of genetics; Christopher Newell (2000), who is a strong voice in the disability lobby and is always concerned with nursing and a philosophy of holism; Nancy Press and her colleagues (2000), who have written specifically about the fears aroused in women by media hype over mutations in two genes associated with breast cancer; and Young-Rhan Um (2000), who described instances in Korea of women who sued for the 'wrongful life' of their handicapped babies.

The argument is made that nurses and midwives are not directly involved in anything to do with genetics, and that the whole field is largely the province of science. However, this is a rapidly changing area of study and application, and all nurses will before long be caring for patients who receive treatments based on genetics and genetically modified human and/or animal tissue. Nurses and midwives need to ask about and face up to some fundamental issues about genetics and care, and indeed the future of life generally, in health care, economics, politics and management.

Dolly, the cloned sheep, was greeted with equal degrees of joy and apprehension in 1996. By 2002 she had developed arthritis and scientists were concerned that this could be related to the cloning process. However, by then she was one among hundreds of cloned sheep, cows and pigs waiting in various laboratories to be used for further research. The five piglets that made news on Christmas day 2002 are potentially the parents of herds of pigs whose organs could be used for transplanting into humans. 'Demand for organs for transplants far outstrips the supply of human tissue, but the use of animal organs in humans is controversial because some medical experts believe that it could unleash serious diseases' (Court 2002, pp. 1, 4).

Scientific advances fascinate and frighten people in similar measure. At present we find it difficult to give answers to questions that make us look into the future, but asking the questions may at least be an important activity.

- Should we make people in our own image?
- Genetically modified cells may pass on to future generations the alterations to the germ line thus manipulated. The long-term implications are not yet foreseeable.
- It may be possible to alter people's behaviour genetically, especially violence or aggression. Who decides what are the bases for such decisions?

- If a child suffered from an aggressive or violent condition, can a parent give consent to modify the child's behaviour genetically?
- What would be considered to be a 'disease' or not? Is being of small stature a disease?
- Society may need to consider its relationship with disease generally in the light of the possibilities. Even if we could eliminate disease, death would still exist.
- Issues of mental health may play a large role here. Can mental health problems be eliminated? Should they be? Which conditions should be seen as undesirable and/or unwanted? Would that make humankind healthier?
- What other conditions should similarly be genetically removed, and which should not?
- If there was a choice between eliminating one potential condition or disease, but not others, which should it be? On what basis?
- Lifestyle choices may be easier. What would be acceptable and what would not? Who would or should decide?
- Sex selection is already well practised; to what extent should it be controlled? By whom? On what basis?
- Just as wheat can be modified to be sterile (the 'terminator' gene), people may be modified to be sterile. The Nazi experiments in eugenics may have been no more than trial runs.
- Do these possibilities add to human happiness, peace, or stability?
- Even if the possibilities of germ-line therapy prove safe and necessary, can we therefore say they are the right ones? While human and animal organ transplants are being considered, other more mechanical approaches are also tried. Which may be better, or more right?
- There is potential for abuse in all experiments and it may be difficult to make claims against manufacturers or surgeons when problems arise years later.
- Insurance companies may want to stipulate who they will cover and who not. Discrimination may be a serious possibility.

Other less potentially devastating treatments and scientific advances have, however, been no less controversial and ethically challenging. Fetal tissue transplants for patients suffering from

Parkinson's disease (Bain 1993), in-vitro fertilisation for postmenopausal women (Chalmers 1994), posthumous parenthood (Klotzko 1998a), and pre-implantation genetic diagnosis (Klotzko 1998b) are some instances of possible life-saving procedures; in most, at least they enhance quality of life. Although it is never easy to determine quality of life, at least we should nevertheless respect other people's opinions. We are faced, however, with the big quandary:

- Just because some treatment, machine, or medication is available, does it mean that we should use it?
- In health care generally, the easiest word for a long time has been 'yes'. When may it be necessary or ethically preferable to say 'no'?

We may need to ask ourselves much more thoroughly than we have done so far what kind of life we want to lead and pass on to our offspring, and how and why. The voice of nursing is vital if this debate is to be applicable generally.

SPIRITUALITY

Perhaps it is not surprising that spirituality has come to have a more prominent place in nursing. Micro and macro events have led to alienation in many areas of life and nurses, as well as many other professionals, have to make sense of what is happening to them. Many people are beginning to experience a need to 'connect' again and are becoming aware of the spiritual aspects of all life as a means for connecting.

Finding a realistic definition of spirituality is almost impossible. By its very essence, it cannot be tied to any one thing. Margaret Fuller and Tom Strong (2001) have suggested three possible expressions of aspects of spirituality:

1. *Spirituality is what we do with the fire inside us, about how we channel our eros.*
2. *Spirituality is something beyond, or greater than, ourselves.*
3. *Spirituality is a meaningful or sacred sense of connectedness in diverse relationships, comparable to Buber's* [see Ch. 1] *I–Thou relationships* (p. 201).

The sense of being connected with all things, or needing to connect, is thus a very important aspect. This concerns in particular the connections with people, but also with nature, and indeed all living things. It is not simply something 'beyond' or other-worldly that is occasionally invoked, but something that IS, that needs to be acknowledged.

For many people the fact of becoming ill is a moment of needing to question their existence. Nurses are not unfamiliar with the hard questions asked at such times. They may not be able to give any answers but, in their relationships with patients and clients, they are present and witness the struggles. The aspects of receptivity, relatedness and responsiveness of an ethic of care are thus strongly evident. The relationship on which nursing is based is also a 'partnership, in which respect for patients and for their values and beliefs is a leading ethical force' (Cohen et al 2001, p. 33).

Spirituality is not necessarily related to religion, although religious practices may be part of spiritual understanding.

Many patient care plans include asking about religious affiliation, but they may not be yet be ready to take spiritual aspects into account. Cynthia Cohen and colleagues (2001) suggest that very general questions could be asked that convey empathy and may not be difficult to answer. 'What are your sources of support when you are ill?' or 'Name and describe your spiritual belief system', may be means of understanding patients better and may lead to further discussion without being intrusive (p. 34).

The alienation that many nurses experience is caused by various factors. Increasing use of technology decreases direct physical contact with patients, as does the greater time spent in documentation. Patients have shorter stays in hospitals and there is less of a chance to get to know them well. The pace of life in general encourages more fleeting relationships. Nurses move between jobs more frequently, becoming less attached to patients and colleagues. Specialist nurses may be working more on their own rather than in teams.

The pace of life in general is quicker, and in towns people may be hardly aware of what is happening around them in nature. Our gardens no longer supply our food, and air travel takes us to far-away places in a short time, making it unnecessary to confront the forces of rivers and mountains. Television removes us from the actual suffering of the people we see. A kind of clinical cleanliness is over much of what really happens in the world and us. The distance thus caused may be large or small, experienced or metaphorical, but it is real. It is not unreasonable that people feel strongly that they need to reconnect with the 'real' world around them.

At the same time, the very means that have alienated people also provide sources for reconnecting: television and the Internet enable them to access and know many different approaches to spirituality, from the very ancient to the very modern. Perhaps more than any other subject, the world of the spirit (the Greek and Hebrew word for spirit is the same as for wind) cannot be captured. Nurses who come into contact with people who express spirituality, or are themselves engaged in practices or searching for understanding, will be aware that respect and openness may be the best attitude to cultivate, to receive what is offered without judgement. Only in this way can a dialogue be created that may lead to insight and analysis.

Spirituality has much to do with experience and how this is expressed. David Brandon (2000) is one among many who have written about their experiences of neglect and abuse as children and who have later used the experience to help others. This has led them to connect with people in similar circumstances, and to turn a negative event or part of life into something positive. Such ways of using what is given and seeing it in a greater perspective, or using it for good, is in itself a spiritual practice. Working with what is there means accepting what is given but transcending it not just for personal gain, but for the wider good. That is also an ethical act. Thus, spirituality and ethics have much in common.

Great numbers of books are available about many aspects of spirituality and health care. A number of journals are also concerned with nursing in particular, such as *Sacred Space*, and with pastoral and health care more generally, such as *Contact*. An internet search will quickly give readers information on other printed material in their field of interest.

INTERNATIONAL NURSING ETHICS

Although nursing may be a world-wide profession and its technical work is similar everywhere, its experience is far from similar. Because culture varies not only from country to country but from locality to locality, ethical understanding may also vary.

Anne Davis (1999) has tried to comprehend why American and UK nursing has had such a profound influence on countries in

Asia, Africa, South America and indeed in other areas of the world. She believes that this is due in part to the early American academic nursing lead, that English had become the dominant international language, and that both American and UK nurses travel widely. In the process, American and UK values were also transported, in particular the values of self-reliance, individualism and informed consent. Gradually, however, these values came to be seen as too culturally exclusive. Indeed, local culture and values have something to offer that may be more appropriate locally, and may also teach American and UK nursing and nurses (and others) that their cultural voice is different but no less important and valid.

Davis (1999) believes that there are broadly two different types of culture world-wide. In a collectivist culture, loyalties of individuals to a group, such as the family or clan, outweigh individual rights. Most of these are found in Asian, African and South American countries and constitute about 70% of all cultures. However, 'Individualist cultures, in which the rights of the individual are central and must be balanced with notions of the common good, tend to be more limited to North America and Europe' (p. 123). Thus, Davis asks,

- '[A]re there ethical notions of caring, ethical principles and virtues, that could be endorsed as true for all nurses everywhere?' (p. 123).

She herself replies by saying that some would answer with 'yes' and others with 'no'.

It has often been said that, just as a butterfly flapping its wings over Tokyo will affect the weather in London, so what a nurse does in the most remote part of the world affects what nurses do in the most sophisticated hospitals anywhere in the world, and vice versa. Through personal contacts and the media we know of each other and depend on each other much more than we may realise. Little can be said or written today that is not influenced by people from very different countries and cultures. The global village is here to stay. This connectedness is also an emotional and spiritual tool. Journals such as *Nursing Ethics* can be nothing other than international; it is the dialogue created in the pages of such journals that informs practice and theory. More than any other means, international ethical dialogue furthers ethical practice itself.

Postscript

On the wall over my desk I have a note with the sentence 'All ethics is a training in sympathy'. I do not remember who said or wrote it, but it is a good reminder of what ethics is about. Perhaps I would more easily use 'empathy' instead of 'sympathy', however. Trying to understand the world of other persons, and to respond in such a way that they know that they have been understood, really does sum up the practice of ethics.

The subtitle of this book 'the caring relationship' epitomises largely what I am trying to convey. Any relationship is important, and we are shaped and influenced by the person or group we are with; we also shape and influence that person or group. We cannot help doing that, but how we do it matters. I am increasingly concerned that we should respect one another. To see another person simply as the person he or she is, value that person simply for being that person, and be with that person as honestly as we can, is not always easy, but it is always enriching for all concerned. Ethical challenges will always throw us into situations in which we are unsure, vulnerable, and perhaps quite paralysed with fear, maybe acting contrary to our normal character. 'Doing something' may not always be the best solution, but 'being with' always is. As nurses we may witness many more ethical dilemmas than we may ever experience ourselves. We learn a great deal from life's problems, but not until we actually experience a situation do we know how we would act and react, and what we value about it. Having had to be with others in their moments of challenge and stress will nevertheless have been a 'school in sympathy'. From sympathy grows empathy. So my quote is perhaps right after all: sympathy needs to come first, but being empathic is also being ethical in the best way we can.

References

Aiken L 1998 Powerful nurses protecting patients. Nursing Standard 13 (7): 30-31

Akid M 2001a For nurses and patients, it's a matter of life and death. Nursing Times 97 (12): 11

Akid M 2001b Guidelines for nursing care on the cards [news]. Nursing Times 97 (50): 8

Albarran J W 1995 Should nurses be politically aware? British Journal of Nursing 4 (8): 461-465

Allen C 1992 Ode to Joy. Nursing Times 88 (10): 24

Allison A, Ewens A 1998 Tensions in sharing client confidences while respecting autonomy: implications for interprofessional practice. Nursing Ethics 5 (5): 441-450

Amnesty International 1997 Nurses and human rights (AI index: ACT 75/20/97) Amnesty International, London

Anderson G 2000 Nursing, ethics and genetics: calling for a multiplicity of voices in our ethical discourse [editorial]. Nursing Ethics 7 (3): 187-189

Anderson G W, Monsen R B, Rorty M V 2000 Nursing and genetics: a feminist critique moves us towards transdisciplinary teams. Nursing Ethics 7 (3): 191-204

Anonymous 1987 Law report: sterilisation of mentally retarded girl is authorised. Bulletin of Medical Ethics (26): 7-9

Anonymous 1990 Law report: US Supreme Court defends right to die. Bulletin of Medical Ethics (60): 23-24

Anonymous 1998 Kiss and hell. Nursing Times 94 (5): 36-37

Anonymous 1999 'We went through psychological hell': a case report of prenatal diagnosis. Nursing Ethics 6 (3): 250-252

Anonymous 2000a Nurses warn against euthanasia move [news]. Nursing Times 96 (5): 10

Anonymous 2000b Whose power, whose ethics? A student nurse's narrative. Nursing Ethics 7 (1): 63

Anonymous 2000c Dilemmas. Nursing Times 96 (6): 31

Anonymous 2001a Screening embryos [news]. Bulletin of Medical Ethics (169): 11

Anonymous 2001b Medical treatment at the end of life [news]. Bulletin of Medical Ethics (166): 5

Anonymous 2001c Dear Nurse. Nursing Times 97 (28): 29

Arras J D 1998 A case approach. In: Kuhse H, Singer P (eds) A companion to bioethics. Blackwell, Oxford, p 106-114

Asplund K, Britton M 1990 Do-not-resuscitate orders in Swedish medical wards. Journal of Internal Medicine 228: 139-145. In: Schultz L 1997 Not for resuscitation: two decades of challenge for nursing ethics and practice. Nursing Ethics 4 (3): 227-238

Audit Commission 2001 Online. Available: http://www.audit-commission.gov.uk

Baillie L 1996 How nurses view emotional involvement with patients. Nursing Times 92 (9): 35-36

Bain L 1993 Fetal transplantation in Parkinson's disease. British Journal of Nursing 2 (20): 1012-1016

Barr O 1997 Euthanasia: the wider social context [letter]. British Journal of Nursing 6 (17): 1015

Beauchamp T L, Childress J F 2001 Principles of biomedical ethics, 5th edn. Oxford University Press, New York

Begley A-M 2000 Preparation for practice in the new millennium: a discussion of the moral implications of multifetal pregnancy reduction. Nursing Ethics 7 (2): 99-112

Benjamin M, Curtis J 1986 Ethics in nursing, 2nd edn. Oxford University Press, New York

Benner P, Wrubel J 1989 The primacy of caring. Addison Wesley, Menlo Park, CA

Berggren I, Severinsson E 2000 The influence of clinical supervision on nurses' moral decision making. Nursing Ethics 7 (2): 124-133

Bernat J L 1998 A defense of the whole-brain concept of death. Hastings Center Report 28 (2): 14-23

Binnie A 1998 How to grow more leaders. Nursing Times 94 (28): 24-25

Birtwistle J, Nielsen A 1998 Do not resuscitate: an ethical dilemma for the decision-maker. British Journal of Nursing 7 (9): 543-549

Bishop A, Scudder J 1996 Nursing ethics: therapeutic caring presence. Jones and Bartlett, Boston, MA

Boyd K 1997 Deontology. In: Boyd K M, Higgs R, Pinching A J (eds) The new dictionary of medical ethics. BMJ Publishing, London, p 68

Brandon D 2000 Bringing spirituality into care planning. Care Plan 7 (1): 9-11

Breier-Mackie S 2001 Patient autonomy and medical paternity: can nurses help doctors to listen to patients? Nursing Ethics 8 (6): 510-521

Brinchmann B S 2000 'They have to show that they can make it': vitality as a criterion for the prognosis of premature infants. Nursing Ethics 7 (2): 141-147

British Medical Association 1995 Advance statements about medical treatments. London: BMA. Online. Available: http://www.bma.org.uk/ethics

British Medical Association 1999 Withholding and withdrawing life-prolonging medical treatment; guidance for decision making. BMJ Books, London

Buber M 1937 I and Thou. (Trans Smith R G 1958, latest impression 1996) T and T Clark, Edinburgh

Buxton V 1996 Signs of the times. Nursing Times 92 (38): 29

Cain P 1997 Using clients. Nursing Ethics 4 (6): 465-471

Cain P 1998 Comment. Nursing Ethics 5(4): 368-369

Callahan D 1993 Pursuing a peaceful death. Hastings Center Report 23 (4): 33-38

Cameron M E, Schaffer M, Park H-A 2001 Nursing students' experience of ethical problems and use of ethical decision-making models. Nursing Ethics 8 (5): 432-445

Campbell A V 1984a Moderated love. SPCK, London

Campbell A V 1984b Moral dilemmas in medicine, 3rd edn. Churchill Livingstone, Edinburgh

Carlisle D 1996 Errors but not trials. Nursing Times 92 (42): 50-51

Castledine G 1997 Whistleblowing guidelines for nursing colleagues. British Journal of Nursing 6 (11): 654

Castledine G 2000 Clinical governance: opportunity for nurses? British Journal of Nursing 9 (10): 670

Castledine G 2001a Euthanasia: what is the nursing and medical role? British Journal of Nursing 10 (8): 550

Castledine G 2001b A&E nurse who physically and racially abused patients. British Journal of Nursing 10 (8): 490

Castledine G 2001c It is possible to recognise higher level nurses. British Journal of Nursing 10 (12): 822

Chalmers C 1994 Fertility and the menopause. British Journal of Nursing 3 (9): 450-453

Chamberlain M 2001 Human rights education for nursing students. Nursing Ethics 8 (3): 211-222

Chambliss D F 1996 Beyond caring. Hospitals, nurses, and the social organization of ethics. University of Chicago Press, Chicago, IL

Charnock A 2001 Who's afraid of clinical governance? Nursing Times 97 (50): 34-35

Churchill L 1977 Ethical issues of a profession in transition. American Journal of Nursing 77 (5): 873-875

Clarke J, O'Neill C S 2001 An analysis of how The Irish Times portrayed Irish nursing during the 1999 strike. Nursing Ethics 8 (4): 350-359

Cohen C B, Wheeler S E, Scott D A, and the Anglican Working Group in Bioethics 2001 Walking a fine line: physician inquiries into patients' religious and spiritual beliefs. Hastings Center Report 31 (5): 29-39

Cook M J 2001 The renaissance of clinical leadership. International Nursing Review 48: 38-46

Court M 2002 These five little piggies lead the race for the £5bn organ transplant market. The Times 3 Jan p 1 (col 1-8), p 4 (col 1-2)

Craig K 2001 The question of choice. Nursing Times 97 (41): 12

Crispi F, Crisci C 2000 Patients in persistent vegetative state ... and what of their relatives? Nursing Ethics 7 (6): 533-534

Crouch D 2001 Caught between a rock and a hard place. Nursing Times 97 (49): 24-25

Curtin L L 1979 The nurse as advocate: a philosophical foundation for nursing. Advances in Nursing Science 1 (3): 1-10

Cutliffe J 1999 Health care should be rationed. British Journal of Nursing 8 (5): 276

Cutliffe J R and Proctor B 1998 An alternative training approach to clinical supervision: 1. British Journal of Nursing 7 (5): 280, 282-285

Cutliffe J R, Epling M, Cassidy P et al 1998a Ethical dilemmas in clinical supervision 1: need for guidelines. British Journal of Nursing 7 (15): 920-923

Cutliffe J R, Epling M, Cassidy P et al 1998b Ethical dilemmas in clinical supervision 2: need for guidelines. British Journal of Nursing 7 (16): 978-982

Dalai Lama 1999 Ancient wisdom, modern world. Ethics for a new millennium. Little, Brown, London

David A 2001 The who's who of advanced practice. Nursing Times 97 (45): 29

Davis A J 1999 Global influence of American nursing: some ethical issues. Nursing Ethics 6 (2): 118-125

Davis A J, Aroskar M A, Liaschenko J et al 1997 Ethical dilemmas and nursing practice, 4th edn. Appleton and Lange, Stamford, CT

Dawood M, James J 2001 What are you afraid of? Nursing Times 97 (40): 24-25

Dempski K M 2001 Informed consent - Part 1. In: Killion S W, Dempski K M Legal and ethical issues (Quick Look Nursing). Slack, Thorofare, NJ, p 42-43

Department of Health 1992 The patient's charter. DoH, London

Department of Health 1994 Being heard. The report of a review committee on NHS complaints procedures (the Wilson Report). DoH, London

Department of Health 1995 The patient's charter and you. DoH, London

Department of Health 1998 The new NHS; modern, dependable [executive summary]. DoH, London

Department of Health 2002 Code of conduct for NHS managers. Available at: www.doh.gov.uk/codeofconductconsultation/consult/pdf

Dimond B 1999a Patients' rights, responsibilities and the nurse, 2nd edn. Quay Books, Salisbury

Dimond B 1999b Confidentiality 2: disclosure of information in the public interest. British Journal of Nursing 8 (10): 687-688

Dimond B 2001a Legal aspects of nursing, 3rd edn. Pearson Education, Oxford

Dimond B 2001b Legal aspects of consent 11: compulsory caesarean sections. British Journal of Nursing 10 (15): 1002-1004

Dimond B 2001c Legal aspects of consent 15: living wills and the common law. British Journal of Nursing 10 (19): 1256-1258

Dimond B 2001d Legal aspects of consent 16: statutory provisions and living wills. British Journal of Nursing 10 (20): 1327-1329

Dimond B 2001e Legal aspects of consent 17: not for resuscitation instructions. British Journal of Nursing 10 (21): 1392-1394

Dixon N 1998 On the difference between physician-assisted suicide and active euthanasia. Hastings Center Report 28 (5): 25-29

DuBose E R, Hamel R, O'Connell L J 1994 A matter of principles? Ferment in US bioethics. Trinity Press International, Valley Forge, PA

Duncan A S, Dunstan G R, Welbourne R B (eds) 1981 Dictionary of Medical Ethics, 2nd edn. Darton, Longman and Todd, London

Edgar A 1994 The value of codes of conduct. In: Hunt G (ed) Ethical issues in nursing. Routledge, London, p 148-163

Edgar A, Salek S, Shickle D et al 1998 The ethical QALY. Ethical issues in healthcare resource allocations. Euromed Communications, Haslemere

Eliot T S 1944 Four Quartets, 9th impression 1976. Faber and Faber, London, p 29

Ersoy N and Göz F 2001 The ethical sensitivity of nurses in Turkey. Nursing Ethics 8 (4): 299-312

Frais A 2001 Whistleblowing heroes - boon or burden? Bulletin of Medical Ethics 170: 13-17

Frank A 1989 The diary of a young girl. Trans Massotty S. Penguin, London

Frankena W 1973 Ethics, 2nd edn. Prentice Hall, Englewood Cliffs, NJ

Frankl V 1962 Man's search for meaning. Pocket Books, New York

Fry S 1989 The role of caring in nursing ethics. Hypatia 4 (2): 88-103. Reproduced in: Holmes HB and Purdy LM (eds) Feminist perspectives in medical ethics. Indiana University Press, Bloomington, IN, p 93-106

Fuller M, Strong T 2001 Inviting passage to new discourse: 'Alive moments' and their spiritual significance. Counselling and Psychotherapy Research 1 (3): 200-214

Gillan J 1999 Nurses are sick of being abused. Nursing Times 95 (16): 22

Gillan J 2001 Nurse education needs a lifeline. Nursing Times 97 (49): 31

Gilligan C 1982 In a different voice; psychological theory and women's development. Harvard University Press, Cambridge, MA

Gillon R 1986 Philosophical medical ethics. Wiley, Chichester

Gillon R 1997 Autonomy. In: Boyd K M, Higgs R, Pinching A J (eds) The new dictionary of medical ethics. BMJ Publishing Group, London, p 19-20

Glover D 1999 Self-regulation: apply within. Nursing Times 95 (43): 30-31

Gordon S 1996 Feminism and caring. In: Gordon S, Benner P, Noddings N (eds) 1996 Caregiving. Readings in knowledge, practice, ethics, and politics. University of Pennsylvania Press, Philadelphia, PA, p 256-277

Greipp M E 1995 Culture and ethics: a tool for analysing the effects of biases on the nurse-patient relationship. Nursing Ethics 2 (3): 211-221

Gulley S 1999 Dealing with the dilemmas of confidentiality. Nursing Times 95 (1): 50-51

Haegert S 2000 An African ethic for nursing? Nursing Ethics 7 (6): 492-502

Han S-S, Ahn S-H 2000 An analysis and evaluation of student nurses' participation in ethical decision making. Nursing Ethics 7 (2): 113-123

Harris J 1987 QUALYfying the value of life. Journal of Medical Ethics 13 (3): 117-123

Hayward M 1999 Cardiopulmonary resuscitation: are practitioners being realistic? British Journal of Nursing 8 (12): 810-814

Health Service Ombudsman for England 2000 Annual report. The Stationery Office, London

Henderson V 1964 The Nature of Nursing. American Journal of Nursing 64 (8): 62-68

Heywood Jones I 1999 The UKCC code of conduct; a critical guide. Emap Healthcare, London

Higgs R 1985 Case conference: a father says 'Don't tell my son the truth'. Journal of Medical Ethics 11 (3): 153-158

Hill A P 2000 Protecting the public through self-regulation. British Journal of Nursing 9 (12): 745

Hirschfeld M 2002 Home-based long-term care [interview]. Nursing Ethics 9 (1): 101-104

Hockey L 2002 Interview. Nursing Ethics 9 (2): 122-125

Holmes H B, Purdy L M (eds) 1992 Feminist perspectives in medical ethics. Indiana University Press, Bloomington, IN

Hoose B 1997 Extraordinary and ordinary means. In: Boyd K M, Higgs R, Pinching A J (eds) The new dictionary of medical ethics. BMJ Publishing, London, p 93

Hoskins R 2001 It's our duty to stop racism. Nursing Times 97 (39): 20

Hunt G 1991 Can nursing lead care? Nursing Standard 5 (25): 18

Hunt G 1999 Abortion: why bioethics can have no answer - a personal perspective. Nursing Ethics 6 (1): 47-57

Husted G L, Husted J H 1991 Ethical decision making in nursing. Mosby-Year Book, St Louis, MO

Illich I 1976 Limits to Medicine. Pelican, Harmondsworth

International Council of Nurses 2000 Code of ethics for nurses. ICN, Geneva

Iredale R 2000 Eugenics and its relevance to contemporary health care. Nursing Ethics 7 (3): 205-214

Jameton A 1984 Nursing practice; the ethical issues. Prentice-Hall, Englewood Cliffs, NJ

Jehovah's Witnesses (undated) Lifesaving alliance; conscience, medicine and alternatives to blood [press information pack]. Jehovah's Witnesses, London

Johnston W 1981 The Mirror Mind. Collins, London

Johnstone M-J 1994 Bioethics; a nursing perspective, 2nd edn. Saunders, Marrickville, NSW

Joseph Rowntree Foundation 1997 Changing mortality ratios in local areas of Britain 1950s-1990s (Social Policy Research findings no. 126). JRF, York

Jourard S M 1971 The Transparent Self. Van Nostrand Reinhold, New York

Kalisch B J 1971 Strategies for developing nurse empathy. Nursing Outlook 19 (11): 714-717

Kass L R 1993 Is there a right to die? Hastings Center Report 23 (1): 34-43

Kennedy L 1990 Euthanasia: the good death. Chatto and Windus, London

Kenny C 2000 Everyone makes mistakes. Nursing Times 96 (48): 14-15

Kirk M 2000 Genetics, ethics and education: considering the issues for nurses and midwives. Nursing Ethics 7 (3): 215-226

Klotzko A J 1998a Life after death. Nursing Times 94 (38): 38-39

Klotzko A J 1998b Unnatural selection. Nursing Times 94 (47): 38-39

Klotzko A J 1999 Thy will be done? Nursing Times 95 (8): 42-43

Kopp P 2001 Fit for practice 6.1: what is evidence-based practice? Nursing Times 97 (22): 47-50

Konishi E, Davis A J 2001 The right-to-die and the duty-to-die: perceptions of nurses in the West and in Japan. International Nursing Review 48: 17-28

Kuhse H 1997 Caring: nurses, women and ethics. Blackwell, Oxford

Kuhse H, Singer P 1985 Handicapped babies: a right to life? Nursing Mirror 160 (8): 17-20

Kuhse H, Singer P 1998 What is bioethics? A historical introduction. In: Kuhse H, Singer P (eds) A companion to bioethics. Blackwell, Oxford

le May A 1999 Evidence-based practice (Nursing Times clinical monographs no. 1). Emap Healthcare, London

Lindsay R, Graham H 2000 Relational narratives: solving an ethical dilemma concerning an individual's insurance policy. Nursing Ethics 7 (2): 148-157

Lindseth A 2001 Editorial comment. Nursing Ethics 8 (5): 391-392

Liss P-E, Nordenfelt L 1990 Health care need, values and change: how changed values influence an evaluative concept. In: Jensen U J, Mooney G (eds) Changing values in medical and health care decision making. Wiley, Chichester, p 109-121

London Palliative Care Centre Team 2001 Is Britain ready for voluntary euthanasia? Nursing Times 97 (28): 17

Lord Chancellor's Department 1999 'Making decisions'. The Government's proposals for making decisions on behalf of mentally incapacitated adults. Stationery Office, London

MacInnes D 1999 Ethical issues in clinical research. Nursing Times clinical monograph no. 14. Emap Healthcare, London

MacIntyre A 1985 After virtue, 2nd edn. Duckworth, London

McFall T 2001 Bringing bullies to book. Nursing Times 97 (32): 33

McGauran A 2001 Will 'expert patients' undercut nurses? Nursing Times 97 (39): 12-13

McSherry R, Haddock J 1999 Evidence-based health care: its place within clinical governance. British Journal of Nursing 8 (2): 113-117

Manning R C 1998 A care approach. In: Kuhse H, Singer P (eds) A companion to bioethics. Blackwell, Oxford, p 98-105

Mason S 1997 The ethical dilemma of the do not resuscitation order. British Journal of Nursing 6 (11): 646-649

May W E 1975 Code, covenant or philanthropy. Hastings Center Report 5 (6): 29-38

Mayeroff M 1972 On caring. Harper and Row, New York

Melville M 1997 Consumerism: do patients have power in health care? British Journal of Nursing 6 (6): 337-340

Mill J S 1867 (reprint 1967) Utilitarianism. Longmans, London

Millar B 1997 Honesty on trial. Nursing Times 93 (35): 10-11

Mind (National Association for Mental Health) 2000 The Mind guide to ... advocacy. Mind, London

Morreim E H 1994 Profoundly diminished life: the casualties of coercion. Hastings Center Report 24 (1): 33-42

Morton-Cooper A, Palmer A 2000 Mentoring, preceptorship and clinical supervision; a guide to professional roles in clinical practice, 2nd edn. Blackwell, Oxford

Mulholland H 2001 Whistle down the wind. Nursing Times 97 (31): 12-13

Mulholland H 2002 Ready to advance. Nursing Times 98 (1): 12

Munhall P L 1993 'Unknowing': toward another pattern of knowing in nursing. Nursing Outlook 41 (3): 125-128

Munro R 1999 The innovation game. Nursing Times 95 (4): 62-64

Nahm E-S, Resnick B 2001 End-of-life treatment preferences among older adults. Nursing Ethics 8 (6): 533-543

National Health Service Executive 1999 Making a difference; strengthening the nursing, midwifery and health visiting contribution to health and healthcare. NHS Executive, Leeds

Nelson-Jones R 1982 The theory and practice of counselling psychology. Cassell, London

Newell C 2000 Biomedicine, genetics and disability: reflections on nursing and a philosophy of holism. Nursing Ethics 7 (3): 227-236

Nicholson D 2000 Why honesty is the best policy. Nursing Times 96 (38): 32

Niebuhr H R 1963 The responsible self. Harper and Row, New York

Noble-Adams R 1999 Ethics and nursing research 1: development, theories and principles. British Journal of Nursing 8 (13): 888-892

Noddings N 1984 Caring - a feminine approach to ethics and moral education. University of California Press, Berkeley, CA

Nolan P W, Markert D 2002 Ethical reasoning observed: a longitudinal study of nursing students. Nursing Ethics 9 (3): 243-258

Nolan M, Keady J, Aveyard H 2001 Relationship-centred care is the next logical step. British Journal of Nursing 10 (12): 757

Nouwen H J M, with McNeill D P and Morrison D A 1982 Compassion. Darton, Longman and Todd, London

Nursing and Midwifery Council 2002 Code of professional conduct. NMC, London

Nursing Ethics 1997 4 (4)

Nursing Ethics 2001 8 (3)

Oakley J 1998 A virtue approach to ethics. In: Kuhse H, Singer P (eds) A companion to ethics. Blackwell, Oxford, p 86-97

Oberle K, Singhal N, Huber J et al 2000 Development of an instrument to investigate parents' perceptions of research with newborn babies. Nursing Ethics 7 (4): 327-338

O'Dowd A 1999 UKCC takes tough stance on abuse [news]. Nursing Times 95 (16): 5

Olsen D 2000 The patient's responsibility for optimum healthcare. Disease Management Health Outcomes 7 (2): 57-65

Oppenheimer H 1995 Mattering. Studies in Christian Ethics 8 (1): 60-76

Pattison S 2001 Are nursing codes of practice ethical? Nursing Ethics 8 (1): 5-18

Payne D 2000a Shock study triggers call to ban ageist slurs. Nursing Times 96 (18): 13

Payne D 2000b To die for. Nursing Times 96 (19): 12

Porter M 2002 The duty of care. Radio Times 5-11 Jan, p 14

President's Commission for the Study of Ethical Problems in Medicine and Biomedical and Behavioural Research 1981 Protecting human subjects. The Belmont Report (DHEW publication no. 0578-0012, 1978). US Government Printing Office, Washington, DC

Press N, Fishman J R, Koenig B A 2000 Collective fear, individualized risk: the social and cultural context of genetic testing for breast cancer. Nursing Ethics 7 (3): 237-249

Proctor B 1986 Supervision: a co-operative experience in accountability. In: Marken M, Payne M (eds) Enabling and ensuring. Leicester National Youth Bureau and Council for Education and Training in Youth and Community Work, Leicester

Rankin-Box D 2000 Is there a rational basis underlying alternative medicine? Nursing Times 96 (23): 18

Raths L E, Harmin M, Simon S 1966 Values and teaching. Merrill, Columbus, OH

Raymond B 2001 Does clinical governance make any difference to patient care? Nursing Times 97 (16): 15

Reich M R, Wagner A K, McLaughlin T J et al 1999 Pharmaceutical donations by the USA: an assessment of relevance and time-to-expiry. Bulletin of the World Health Organization 77 (8): 675-680

Rickard M, Kuhse H, Singer P 1996 Caring and justice: a study of two approaches to health care ethics. Nursing Ethics 3 (3): 212-223

Roach M S 1992 The human act of caring. A blueprint for the health professions, rev edn. Canadian Hospital Association, Ottawa

Robertson J 1998 Beyond the dependency culture. People power and responsibility. Adamantine Press, Twickenham

Rogers C 1961 On becoming a person. Constable, London

Rowden R 1998 Unleashing the potential. Nursing Times 94 (43): 62-63

Rushmer R 2000 What will it mean to have a flatter team-based NHS structure? British Journal of Nursing 9 (21): 2242-2248

Russell P, Sander R 1998 Palliative care: promoting the concept of a healthy death. British Journal of Nursing 7 (5): 256-261

Sacks J 1990 Reith lectures: 2 The demoralisation of discourse. The Listener 124 (3192): 9-11

Sainio C, Lauri S, Eriksson E 2001 Cancer patients' views and experiences of participation in care and decision making. Nursing Ethics 8 (2): 97-113

Salussolia M 1997 Is advanced nursing practice a post or a person? British Journal of Nursing 6 (16): 928, 930-933

Salvage J 1985 The politics of nursing. Heinemann, Oxford

Salvage J 1990 The theory and practice of the 'new nursing' [occasional paper]. Nursing Times 86 (1): 42-45

Salvage J 2000 Distinctly valuable. Nursing Times 96 (16): 26

Sanders K 2001 New Dutch Bill decriminalises voluntary euthanasia and doctor-assisted suicide. Ethics Bulletin (RCN) Summer, 2

Schultz L 1997 Not for resuscitation: two decades of challenge for nursing ethics and practice. Nursing Ethics 4 (3): 227-238

Scott H 1999 Should children be able to request euthanasia? [editorial]. British Journal of Nursing 8 (16): 1046

Shaha M 1998 Racism and its implications in ethical-moral reasoning in nursing practice: a tentative approach to a largely unexplored topic. Nursing Ethics 5 (2): 139-146

Sheldon T 2001 Showing a little mercy. Nursing Times 97 (17): 10-11

Shotton L 2000 Can nurses contribute to better end-of-life care? Nursing Ethics 7 (2): 134-140

Smith K V 1996 Ethical decision-making by staff nurses. Nursing Ethics 3 (1): 17-25

Snee N 1999 Let's move on up. Nursing Times 95 (1): 35

Snell J 1997 Thinking Pink. Nursing Times 93 (32): 34

Sommerville A 1997 Declarations. In: Boyd K M, Higgs R, Pinching A J (eds) The new dictionary of medical ethics. BMJ Publishing, London, p65-66

Swider S M, McElmurry B, Yarling R R 1985 Ethical decision-making in a bureaucratic context by senior nursing students. Nursing Research 34: 108-112

Teasdale K 1998 Advocacy in health care. Blackwell Science, Oxford

Tharoor S 2001 Are human rights universal? New Internationalist 332: 34-35

Thiroux, J P 1995 Ethics, theory and practice, 5th edn. Prentice-Hall, Englewood Cliffs, NJ

Thompson I A, Melia K, Boyd K 2000 Nursing ethics, 4th edn. Churchill Livingstone, Edinburgh

Thoreau H D 1849 A week on the Concord and Merrimack Rivers: 'Wednesday'. In: Partington A (ed) (1992) The Oxford dictionary of quotations, 4th edn. Oxford University Press, Oxford, p 697

Tomlinson A L 2001 Training God's spies. Developing the imagination in theological formation [occasional paper]. Contact Pastoral Monograph 11

Tronto J C 1993 Moral boundaries. A political argument for an ethic of care. Routledge, New York

Truog, R D 1997 Is it time to abandon brain death? Hastings Center Report, 27 (1): 29-37

Tschudin V 1991 Beginning with awareness [training package]. Churchill Livingstone, Edinburgh

Tschudin V 1997 Nursing as a moral art. In: Marks-Maran D, Rose P (eds) Reconstructing nursing beyond art and science. Baillière Tindall, London, p 64-90

Tschudin V 2001 European experiences of ethics committees. Nursing Ethics 8 (2): 142-151

Tschudin V (ed) 2003 Approaches to ethics: nursing beyond boundaries. Butterworth-Heinemann, Edinburgh

Tschudin V, McGregor R 2001 Ethics and law [open learning package]. University of Surrey, European Institute of Health and Medical Sciences, Guildford

Tschudin V, with Schober J 1998 Managing yourself, 2nd edn. Macmillan, Basingstoke

Tuckett A 1999 Nursing practice: compassionate deception and the Good Samaritan. Nursing Ethics 6 (5): 383-389

Um Y-R 1999 A study of the ethics of induced abortion in Korea. Nursing Ethics 6 (6): 506-514

Um Y-R 2000 A critique of a 'wrongful life' lawsuit in Korea. Nursing Ethics 7 (3): 250-261

United Kingdom Central Council 1992a Code of professional conduct. UKCC, London

United Kingdom Central Council 1992b The scope of professional practice. UKCC, London

United Kingdom Central Council 1996 Guidelines for professional practice. UKCC, London

United Kingdom Central Council 1999a Fitness for practice. The UKCC Commission for Nursing and Midwifery Education. UKCC, London

United Kingdom Central Council 1999b Making the connection - professional self-regulation and clinical governance. Register 27: 5-8

United Kingdom Central Council 2001 Professional self-regulation and clinical governance. UKCC, London

van der Arend A J G, Remmers-van den Hurk C H M 1999 Moral problems among Dutch nurses: a survey. Nursing Ethics 6 (6): 468-482

van Hooft S 1995 Caring. An essay in the philosophy of ethics. University Press of Colorado, Niwot, CO

van Hooft S 2003 Caring and ethics in nursing. In: Tschudin V (ed) Approaches to ethics: nursing beyond boundaries. Butterworth-Heinemann, Edinburgh

Veatch R M 1972 Models of ethical medicine in a revolutionary age. Hastings Center Report 2 (3): 5-7. In: Aroskar M A 1980. Ethics of nurse-patient relationships. Nurse Educator 5 (2): 18-20

Wainwright P 1998 Comment: using clients: a response to Paul Cain. Nursing Ethics 5 (4): 363-368

Watson J, Ray M (eds) 1990 The ethics of care and the ethics of cure; synthesis in chronicity. National League of Nursing, New York

Weale A (ed) 1988 Cost and choice in health care. King Edward's Hospital Fund for London, London

Weir R F, Peters C 1997 Affirming the decisions adolescents make about life and death. Hastings Center Report 27 (6): 29-40

White C 1998 Will the truth still hurt? Nursing Times 94 (28): 17

Whyte A 1997 Fertile ground. Nursing Times 93 (14): 16

Wigens L 1998 Specialist practice and the professional project for nursing. British Journal of Nursing 7 (5): 266-269

Wilkinson J 1997 Developing a concept analysis of autonomy in nursing practice. British Journal of Nursing 6 (12): 703-707

Wilks M 1999 Euthanasia: intent is the key issue not outcome [comment]. British Journal of Nursing 8 (10): 634

Williams C, Kendall L 1998 Tackling strokes. Nursing Times 94 (32): 32-33

Willis J 1999 Courage to change. Nursing Times 95 (21): 34-35

World Health Organization 2001 Declaration of Helsinki. Bulletin of the World Health Organization 79 (4): 373

World Medical Association 2000 Declaration of Helsinki. WMA, Geneva

Wray E 2001 Assisted suicide and human rights. Bulletin of Medical Ethics 172: 18-21

Index